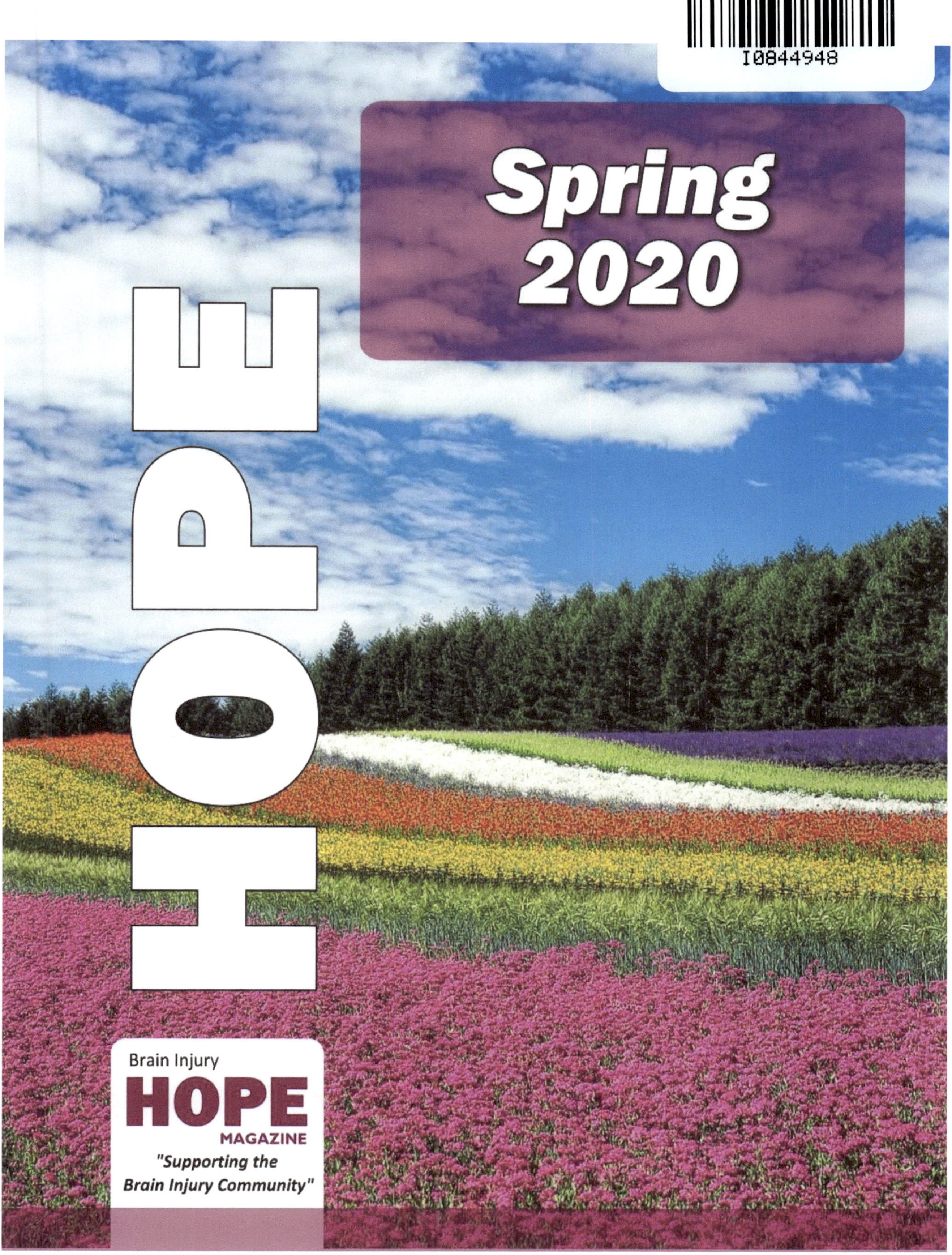
Spring
2020
HOPE
Brain Injury
HOPE
MAGAZINE
"Supporting the
Brain Injury Community"

Welcome

HOPE MAGAZINE

Serving the Brain Injury Community Since 2015

Publisher
David A. Grant

Editor
Sarah Grant

Our Contributors

Marjorie Appleby
Megan Bacigalupo
Stacia Bissell
William Carter
Russ Cobleigh
Rachel Dombeck
Debra Gorman
Nancy Hueber
Ric Johnson
Judith Johnston
Dr. Ted King
Norma Myers
Ralph Poland
Lisa Cohen Ratcliff
James Scott
Carole Starr

Welcome to the Spring 2020 Issue of HOPE Magazine

We've done it now – taken something good and made it even better. Late last year, we announced a big change with HOPE Magazine as we begin the next chapter of our publication as an expanded quarterly magazine.

When Sarah and I first discussed moving to a less frequent, but much larger version of HOPE, there was a lot of excitement. We both knew that this would provide us the opportunity to dig deeper into topics that most help those within the brain injury community.

To that end, our first expanded issue features an in-depth look at how support groups enrich the lives of both survivors as well as those who love them. When we announced a call for support group articles last year, the response was nothing short of heartwarming. Thank you for those who contributed stories for this special section. Your shared experiences will help others as they navigate life after brain injury.

Our next issue will feature a special section about life after brain injury as seen through the eyes of family members and caregivers.

Peace,

David A. Grant
Publisher

Table
of Contents

Spring 2020

Advocacy

Education

Inspiration

Brain Injury
HOPE
NETWORK

Story Callout:
Family Members and Caregivers

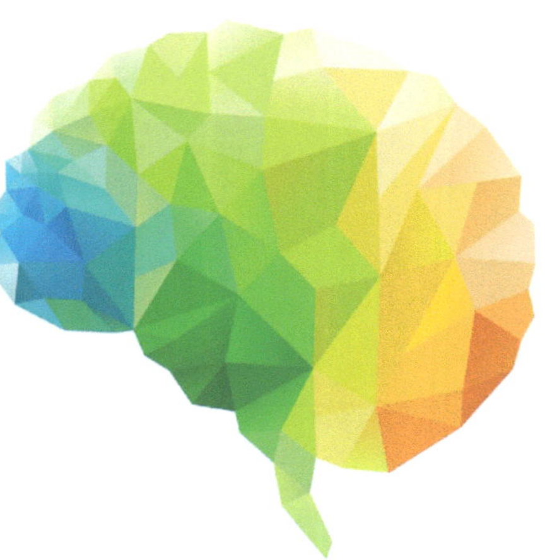

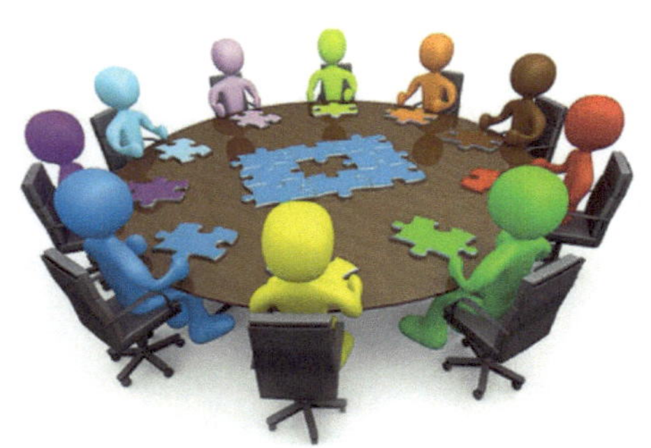

We are looking for stories for the next issue of HOPE Magazine about your experience as a family member or caregiver for someone with a brain injury.

Caregivers and family members face unique challenges when it comes to brain injury of any kind.

Our next issue of HOPE Magazine will be largely dedicated to this important topic.

Your Story has Value!

And now the details...

- We prefer an article length of 800-1,000 words. Longer or shorter pieces will be considered.
- When submitting, please include a photo or photos to be included with your piece.
- Please include 2-3 photos to accompany your submission

Please email your submission to mystory@tbihopeandinspiration.com.

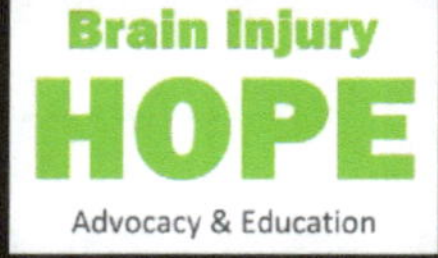

The Porch

By Stacia Bissell

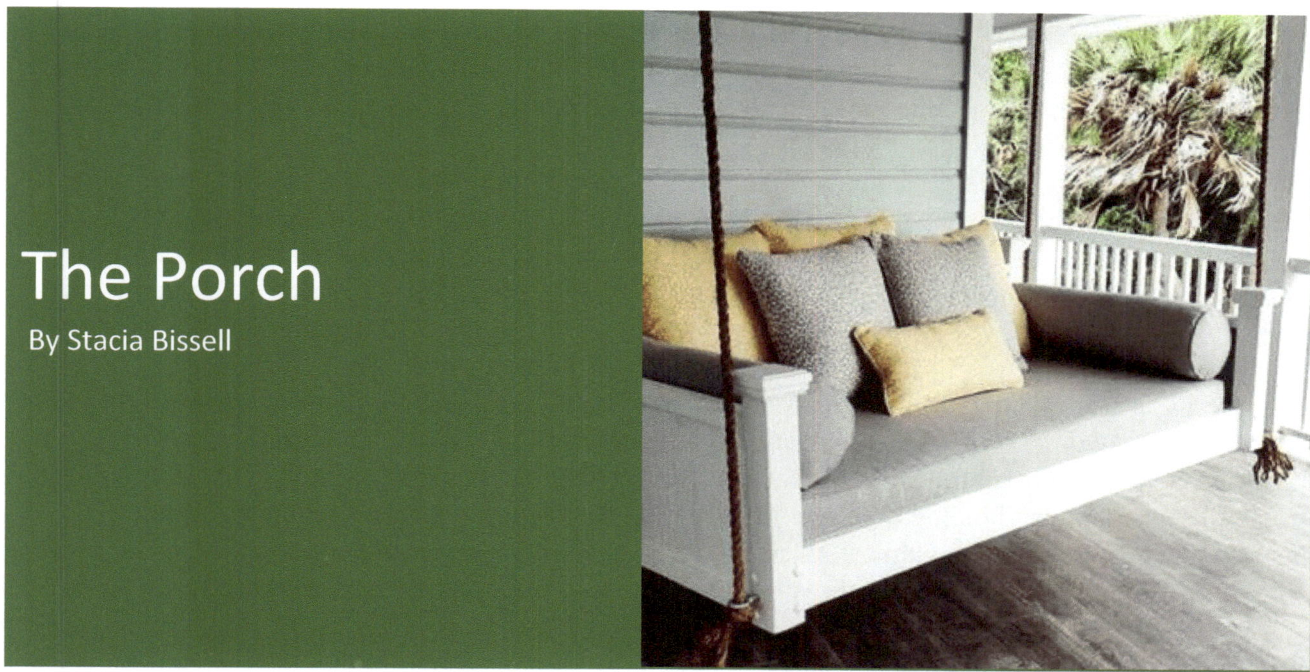

After my *Glass Box* article was published in the January 2018 issue of HOPE magazine, many readers told me they didn't want the story to end with the old me. I called her Version 1.0. I was trapped inside a tightly sealed glass box that was serving as living quarters for my pre-TBI self.

For those unfamiliar with the story, I suffered a traumatic brain injury in September of 2011. At the time, I was married and had three children in their twenties. My social life was robust, and I loved my career in public education. I was a newly licensed middle and high school Principal, and I had just left my job as a math teacher to take on a more administrative role in the middle school where I worked. I had aspirations of running my own school in the near future. My TBI occurred from a bicycle accident that I cannot remember. What I do know is that the moment my helmet hit the pavement, a new version of me began living and breathing. I call her Version 2.0. Simultaneously Version 1.0 was neatly packed away in what I envisioned to be a glass box, and I seemed to lug her around wherever I went. From there, she endlessly teased me, because I could see her and remember her, but did not feel like her. I could not access her with ease, if even at all.

> "What I do know is that the moment my helmet hit the pavement, a new version of me began living and breathing."

My friend Michael responded with, "It does make me want to wrap a porch around your glass box." In his own gentle and insightful way, Michael was suggesting there might be some space that these two versions of me could occupy simultaneously, rather than living separately on each side of the sardonic and unyielding walls.

So I started considering that if the pre-TBI woman in the glass box could step out onto an imaginary porch, and the post-TBI woman I have become could step onto that same porch and have a chat with her, then I might gain some much needed answers for accepting and living life with a brain injury.

What would the two women talk about on that porch? What might each version of me want to say to the other? Would the conversation be relaxing and friendly while they sat in rocking chairs sipping lemonade on Michael's cleverly constructed imaginary porch? Or would awkward or resentful words ensue while they stood facing each other, pondering why the other one was stuck living in the mirror image of the other's body?

Admittedly, it was exciting to entertain the thought of continuing my story at the starting point of the porch, but how would I write about something that couldn't really happen? Usually a precise historian of my own brain injury experiences, I felt I would just be fabricating the next chapter of my story if I loosely created dialog between these two selves to supply readers with more of my narrative. I puzzled over how this would play out and faintly mentioned the porch idea to my friend, Eileen, one day, mainly to continue breathing life into my resolution to connect these two women.

Eileen is a spunky woman in her seventies who sustained a brain injury on the job just hours after my own brain injury occurred. She gently offered that if I trusted her and wanted to, we could set up a time for me to visit her, and she would try bringing me into a light, hypnotic trance to help me draw out some missing pieces. Eileen is a social worker, dance therapist, EMDR specialist, and she's trained in hypnosis and guided imagery. She has worked at world-renowned places like Canyon Ranch and Kripalu as well as maintaining a private practice. I knew I'd be in good hands and gave the idea a green light.

A week later I found myself at Eileen's home sipping tea and exchanging dialog about the prospect of Versions 1.0 and 2.0 meeting on the porch. During our conversation, I also described a peaceful, outdoor place I go to in my mind on the occasions when I meditate. My peaceful place consists of a large plot of bright green ferns bordered by a classic white picket fence with a swinging gate in the front. I discovered this place once as a teen while on horseback with a friend in the wooded mountains near my parents'

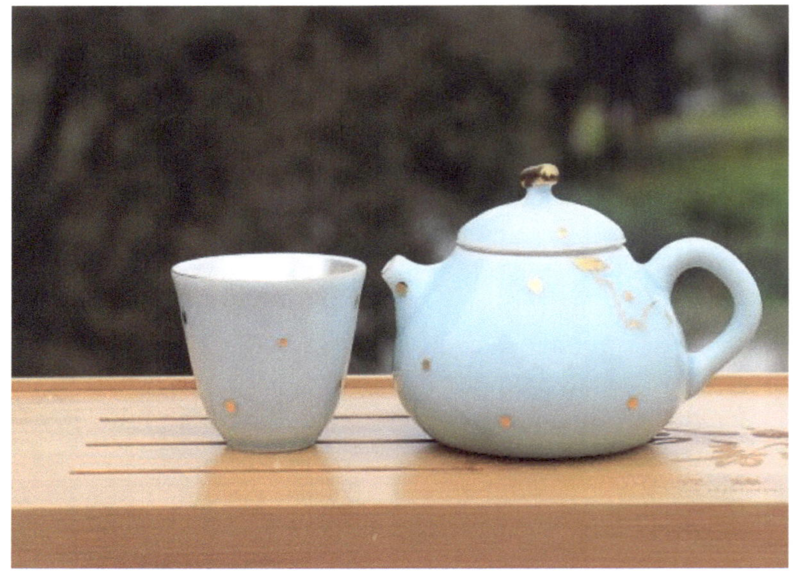

home. I could never find it again, but I always remembered the setting as one of sweet stillness among the tall trees that let filtered sunlight shine through onto the crowded fern patch and the charming white fence that must have outlined someone's estate at one time.

The session began with my lying down on Eileen's couch with my head resting on a soft velour pillow and a creamy warm blanket covering me. With an eye mask over my eyes, my post-TBI auditory sensitivities picked up on the tranquility of Eileen's home and the sound of water faintly dripping from a gutter outside a nearby window. Before long, and with surprisingly little coaxing, Eileen brought me into a deep and relaxed state of mind where I was standing in front of the picket fence surrounding the dense fern patch.

She encouraged me to reach out and open the gate, step through it and close the gate behind me. Without hurrying me, Eileen had me walk peacefully through the soft, cool bed of ferns across to the far side of the lot and asked me to describe what was in front of me. I told her that the fence opened to a clearing in the woods just beyond it. She asked if I could see the glass box anywhere from the edge of the fern patch and then gently prodded me toward it when I told her it was there in the clearing. Before long I was standing in front of the Glass Box.

As if knowing I would arrive today, Version 1.0's quarters already had Michael's front porch fashioned onto it with a set of four or five steps leading up to it. The whole structure was larger than I anticipated it would be, and it hovered off the ground with no real foundation underneath, as if invisible cottage piers were holding it up. Later, when I was out of my trance, I would reflect on whether this generously sized rendition of the glass box raised up high was my way of viewing my pre-TBI self as having a more prominent status than the post-TBI version of me. While this may have been true, it didn't seem healthy or productive to overanalyze it. Besides, I would smile and remember that in my trance state, I had also conjured up a floating glass structure that had no foundation.

From my place on the ground in front of the glass box structure, I could see Version 1.0 calmly sitting in there. I was urged by Eileen to climb up the steps onto the porch and to describe what Version 1.0 looked like. Apparently, I described her as being well groomed and poised, wearing a dark blazer, gray dress pants and black heels. "My typical outfit when I was a schoolteacher," I told her.

When my dissolved marriage was discussed, a trace of tears slowly escaped my eyes and ran down my neck onto the velour pillow beneath my head. Eileen could see that this subject was going to be a hard one for me to face during this session. She checked in with me often to ask what I was looking at or what something felt like physically or emotionally, and carefully asked the right questions to promote dialog between my two selves. At one point Eileen pressed the new me to describe to the old me what is has felt like to be reinvented. She talked about feeling beaten down knowing that friends, family, colleagues and children had pushed the new, more awkward me away. She was downhearted for having a marriage that had stopped working, and she was dispirited by the deep ache that accompanied the loss of the unconcluded career and traditional family she so valued. But even more so, she had a sense of terror wondering if her broken brain had made the wrong decisions about leaving her job and marriage because she may not have thoroughly processed things correctly.

> **"I learned that I *could* trust my post-TBI self to be my own guide."**

While this part of the story sounds somewhat heavy, the silver lining that came from my experience on Michael's porch was that I learned that I could trust my post-TBI self to be my own guide. I could see that I have a resiliency for withstanding life's physical and emotional challenges, and that I have made the correct decisions for my best health and self. I also knew without a doubt that I have the ability to redirect important relationships and to make and sustain meaningful new ones.

When Eileen could detect I was tiring, she brought me back to the clearing in the woods near the fern patch. When she had me focus on the glass box, I realized that I wasn't on the porch any longer. I was standing firmly on the ground. The glass structure with Version 1.0 in it was in the far, far distance, low to the ground, and no more than the size of a postage stamp. Version 1.0 never did step out of the box to meet me on the porch, but the dialog between the women was enough.

I reflected that for years, I had been the brilliant designer of my Version 1.0 life and lived it. Now the memories of it were a beautiful web of artwork. My old life was done, a memory to look back upon as my creative expression set behind the glass of a softer curio cabinet to be cherished. The glass structure, I noted, housed the woman who had once been successful in her multi-tasking roles as wife, mother and educator, but I was ready to let her be a good memory. I was tired of chasing the pieces that prevented Version 2.0 from finding the peace that living in the moment of today was offering.

Version 1.0 no longer holds power over the bold, bright, brave and beautiful person I am today; the woman who has become an advocate, writer and speaker on behalf of the brain injury community. I have learned new skills, traveled more, renewed old relationships, cultivated many new ones, and found interesting and fresh alternatives for spending my leisure time and energy. As my architect friend Michael told me when I shared my visualization experience with him, "You made friends with your psychic image of yourself as an individual in a *Glass Box*, isolated from sensory input, but then by acknowledging that image, it began to lose power over you, it shrank. You let that identity go."

I'm now breaking out Version 3.0. She is arriving!

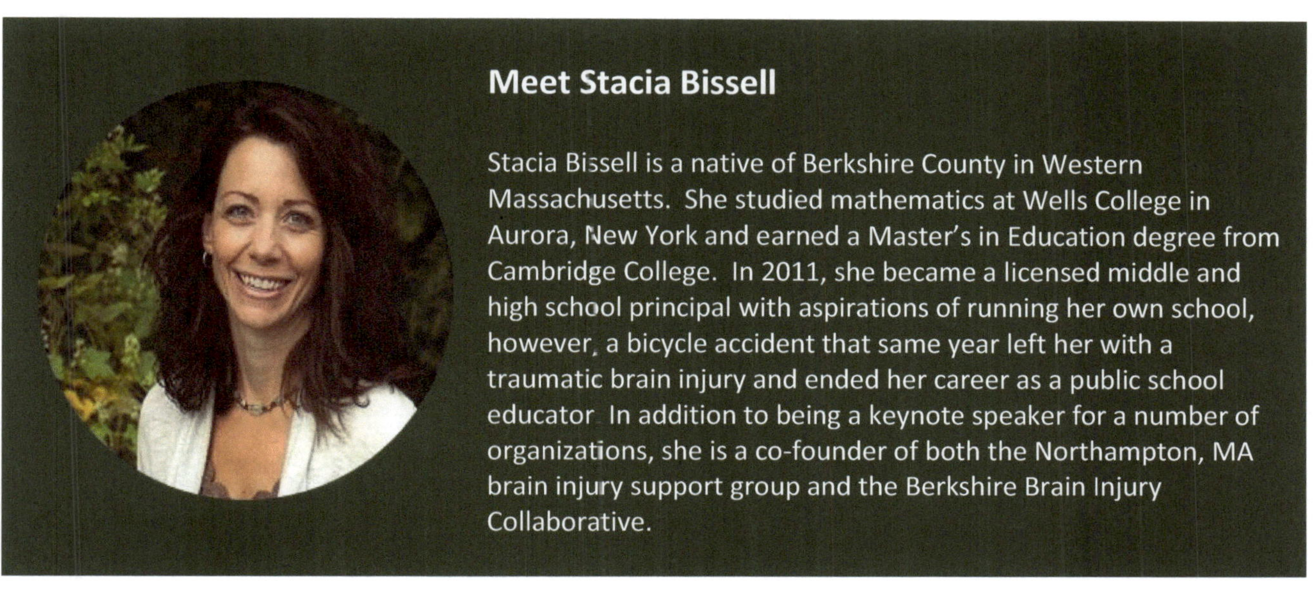

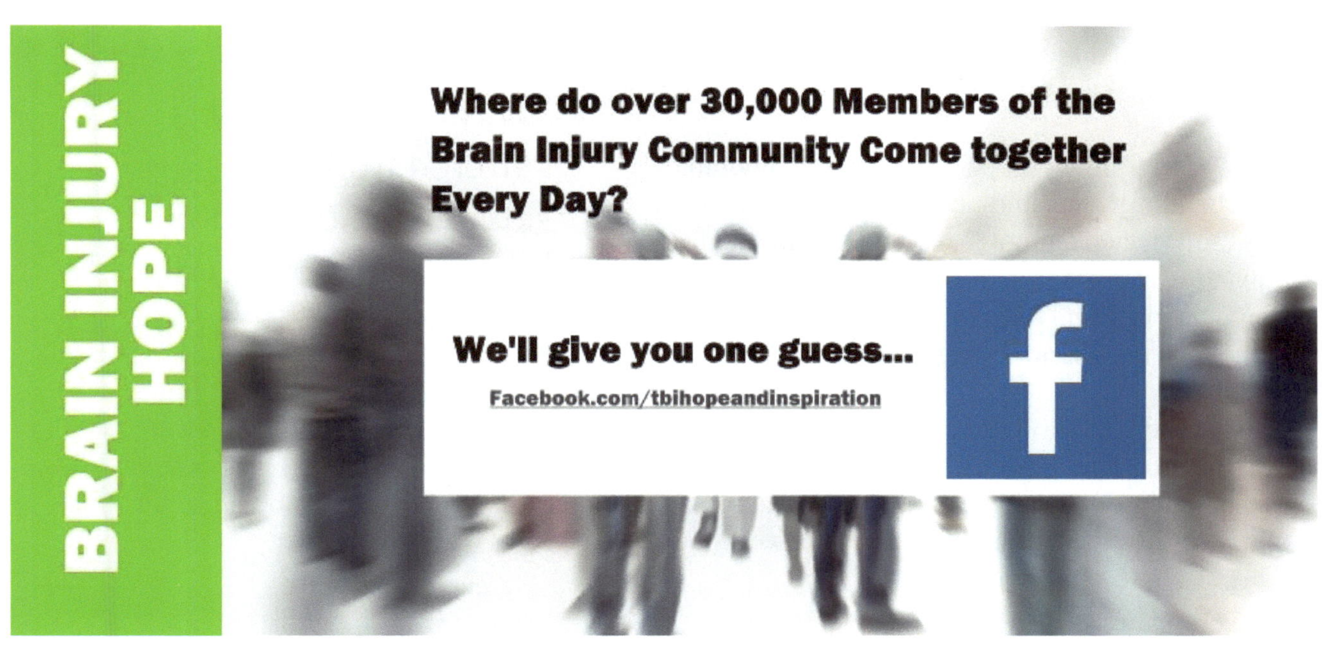

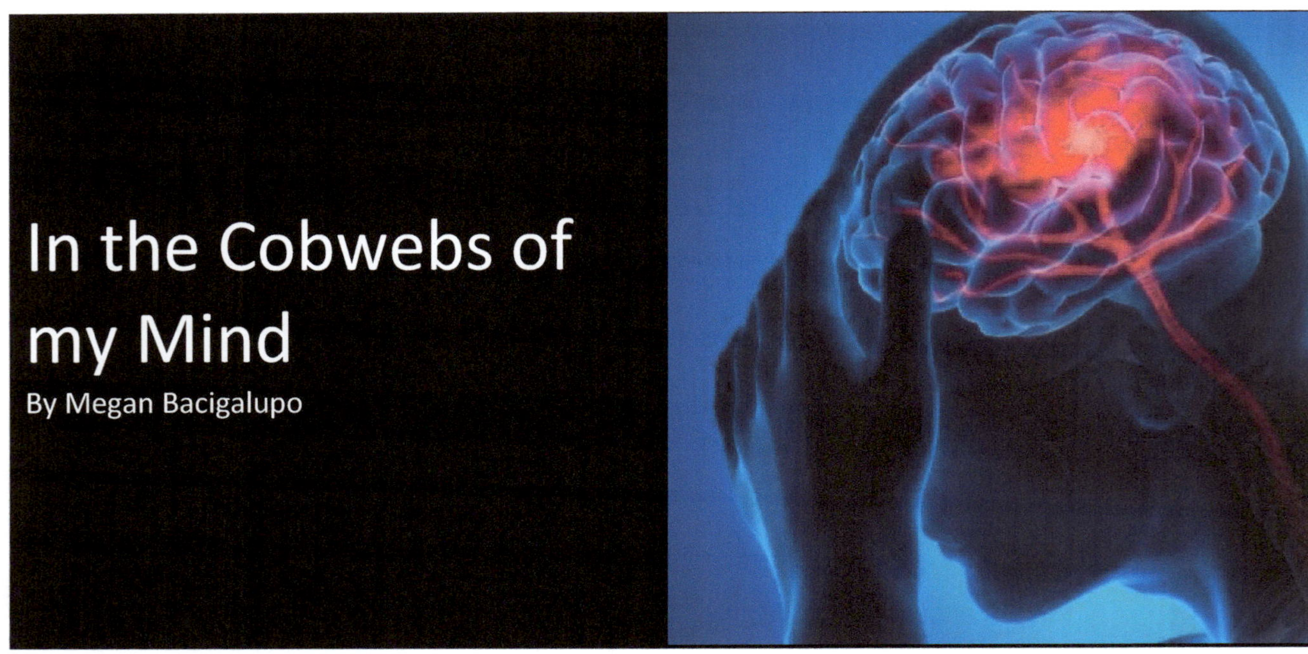

My body became a clock. Time pushed forward as a force moved me to get me to where I needed to go. I felt like a Derby horse with blinders, and all I could see was the ambulance that I imagined — a life source after it was called.

Everything lined up for me almost mathematically the night of September 20, 2017. This was the night I almost died. I was on a city bike in uptown Minneapolis, on my way home. Without warning I suffered from a subarachnoid ruptured brain aneurysm, a brain hemorrhage and stroke.

I heard a whooshing sound in my ears and realized it was coming from inside my head rather than externally. The wheels of the cars around me were turning in sync with the sound in my head. I went partially deaf and then I jumped off the bike. My vision was getting shaky and blurred.

What was to follow was paralyzing pain, a bomb of a headache in my head and neck. It was so unbearable I felt myself detach from it. I was outside my body. Knowing it was not possible to endure this pain, I became helpless and had no choice but to surrender, surrender to the unknown. I gave up control.

> "Without warning I suffered from a subarachnoid ruptured brain aneurysm, a brain hemorrhage and stroke."

In this moment of surrender, a sense of calm came over me. A force was holding me. Aware that the clock was ticking all the while. I guess I was waiting to be rescued. I was lucky I was in front of a coffee shop in my neighborhood. I said to a guy on a cell phone, "Call me an ambulance." At this point I was in shock but still able to function.

I handed off the city bike to someone and a woman sat with me. I heard the sirens and knew they were for me. Still in excruciating pain, I answered the questions the paramedics asked, and they got me in the vehicle. I vomited twice in the ambulance. The next thing I remember was slowly passing out. I remember the sensation of being wheeled out of the ambulance, bouncing, and the rickety noise of the stretcher as I entered the hospital.

My medical records state that I arrived unresponsive and moaning. I also learned from my medical records I had a seizure and was repeating to the medical team that I was going blind. I have no recollection of these last details. I was intubated. Two-part surgery. Coiling the ruptured aneurysm by going up into the brain through the main artery in the groin. And a ventriculostomy. Drilling and cutting open a hole in my skull. They inserted a tube or drain to take the pressure off the brain. My blood mixed with my cerebral spinal fluid hung in a bag on my hospital pole. I was attached to it.

I was in the ICU for two weeks.

My angels and the living dead sat, walked and wandered in a circular motion as they repeatedly passed by my bed with out-stretched arms, almost like they were tempting me or inviting me. They each gave me several chances to leave. I continued to watch them. I never felt that I was to join them. They were good company. This was the welcoming committee. They wanted me to know they were there.

Persistent in their motion and very ghost-like, all of them wore hospital gowns like the one I had on. Their faces were all dark and shadowed, without eyes or features. I was trying to figure out who they were. The one who was always sitting had a silhouette of a huge Beehive hairdo like the one my grandmother wore for years. She was always in the chair next to me and outstretched her arms from time to time.

I somehow made connections as I traveled in two worlds. I knew they were the living dead and my angels. I stretched in my mind to guess who the others might be. Some were dead relatives, and some were angelic. I would wake up or some nurse would wake me and my dead relatives and angels would fade out. I had a sense that they were always near, never far away.

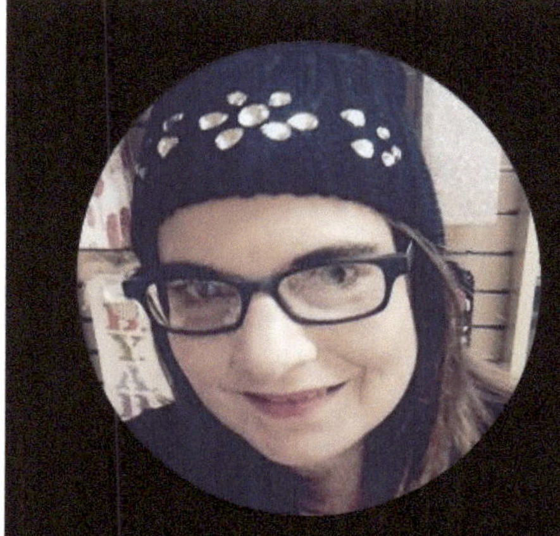

Meet Megan Bacigalupo

Megan Bacigalupo is a sensitive, an empath and intuitive. She has explored many shamanic journeys with the help of her guides. She has always considered herself a solitary eclectic and a seeker. She has a degree in Human Services. Megan is a survivor of a hemorrhagic stroke. She loves to write.

The New Everyday Version of You

By William Carter

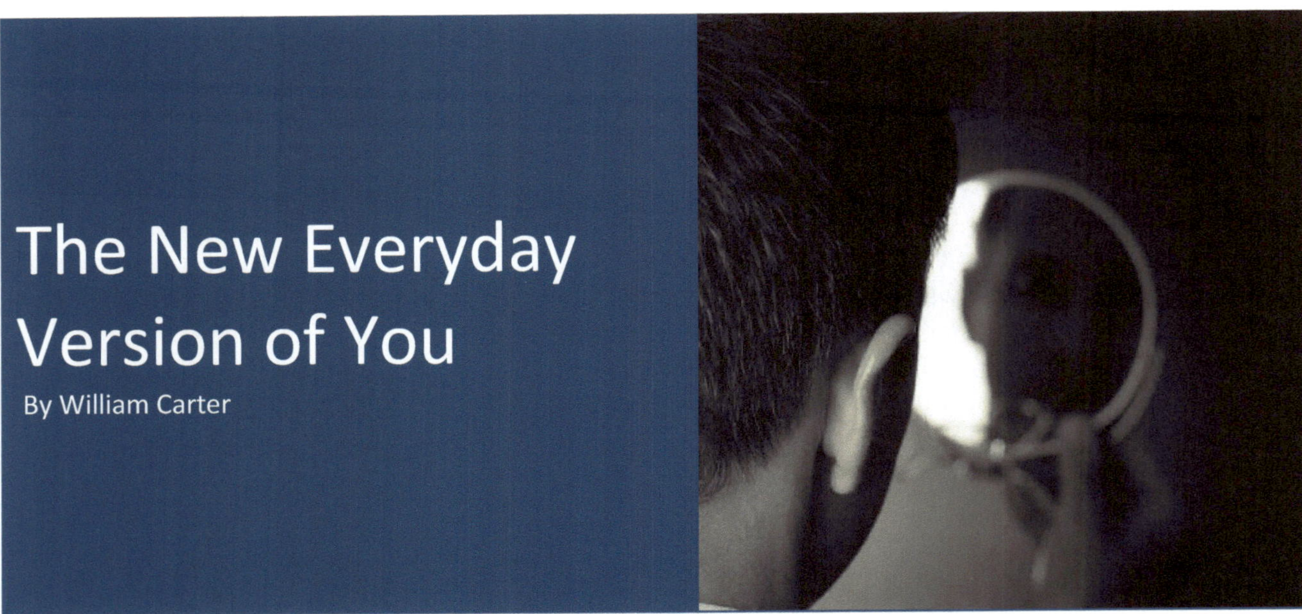

Almost seven months ago, I underwent surgery for a pacemaker at Emory Hospital. I went from having a heartbeat of thirty-five to a heartbeat that measured sixty-five after my surgery. If you want to know what this feels like, it feels like I am a whole new person. I feel like I have a second chance at life.

I should probably explain a few things. I have had to adjust to a new me for a long-time. When I was seventeen years-old, I was driving home from work, when my Honda Accord was involved in a head-on collision with a Suburban. They don't know whether I crossed the line or if the Suburban crossed the line, or if we both did, but the accident resulted in me suffering a collapsed lung, a ruptured spleen, and a traumatic brain injury. My wounds were so severe that I had to be in a coma. Sounds a bit rehearsed, am I right? That's because I have had to give this speech ever since my accident to justify the new me. My mother has told me that the grief of someone with a traumatic brain injury is grieving the loss of who they used to be.

"After suffering a brain injury, there is grief. It looks and feels just like real grief."

I used to be an all-AP student, president of the drama club, member of the debate team, Model UN award winner, playwright, and someone who, at the very least, thought he had a sufficient amount of forward momentum. That was me before, before the accident, before the injury, before I was familiar with the stuttered steps of a post-accident limp, before I knew what it was to struggle to remember the events of the day. Yes, I have grown leaps and bounds. Before the limp, was the cane, and before that, there was the walker, and before that, oh before that, there was the bane of my existence, the dreaded wheelchair. I used to be at the top of the world, and at this point, I felt under it.

After suffering a brain injury, there is grief. It looks and feels just like real grief. It follows the same shape and rhythm, but you can't call it grief out-loud. You're too busy going through the stages. First, there's denial. This injury isn't going to stop me. I am going to get back to where I was before. I am going to walk. I am going to recover. I am going to retake the SAT. That is actually where I was supposed to be the day after my accident. I had been working with a math tutor the whole summer, and I was feeling good. I was going to retake the SAT and get my math score up to the level it needed to be to go to Wake Forest University.

Denial is easy. It's not like the steps that follow after. You just have to tell yourself that what is isn't, and people lie to themselves all the time. "The diet is really going to work this time." "I do deserve this promotion." "I am not that talkative; they don't know what they're talking about." The truth is that I really am that talkative. Denial is a cinch. I am going to get better. This brain injury is like a cold - you get over it. And after enough therapy, I am going to back to normal and good as new. Finishing high-school was hard, but I graduated, didn't I?

I've got this. Denial is easy. Anger is harder.

The anger is the frustration at yourself. The anger is the frustration at your circumstances. "Why can't I just seem to remember this reading?" "Everyone tells me to have fun at college, but I can't do that and have good grades." "Why can't I just do my work faster?" "Why do I have to take so long on every little thing?" "Why can't I drive?" "Why can't I walk better?" "Why do I have to feel like the awkward guy in every single conversation?" They tell me that an injury means I heal. WHY CAN'T I HEAL? But they aren't stages, because you can't stay there. You have to jump back to denial.

Just to keep going, you have to believe that you aren't different. That one day you will be your smart self again. But then, you're still the college freshman waking up at four AM every morning. So, what if I do these exercises? And, what if I ask God every day? What if I read my bible and pray really long and good? I mean, God, what do I need to do? Is there something I can do? And, there is nothing you can do. You can wait, because healing will come.

Like grief over loss, healing will come, but that healing takes far longer, than you have time for. In the moment you are feeling you need healing, and you want God to just give you a little taste, a little sampler, a sip, just to keep going.

You are healing, but it sure looks like that cup that is supposed to overflow is empty and depression sets in. Is this just who I am? Am I simply a tragedy case? The accident is the only good story he's got, Mr. One Hit Wonder. You don't want it, but it hangs over you and haunts you, but you don't even care. Or, at least you tell that to yourself, as you wrap your disappointments and what you think are dashed hopes around you as protection from actually really dealing with this.

Then, not all at once, not like a ton of bricks, not like the lighting from heaven, but with the slow, diligent progress of a tree growing or a baby developing, you find acceptance. This is me. Yes, I have a brain injury, and it has shaped me into who I am today. I can persevere, and I am stronger for it. I am still healing. I am still changing, and every day, I have to accept the me of today.

I have to move on from the me of yesterday, stop placing all the hope on the me of tomorrow, and accept and love the me of today. Brain injury or not, this is the daily battle of us all. I am not who I was. I am not yet who I will be. Today, I am. And that is good enough.

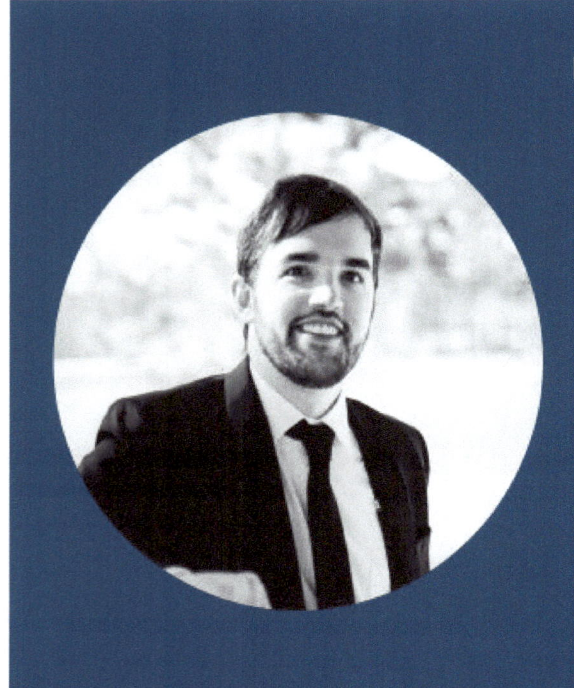

Meet William Carter

Will Carter is a native of Roswell, Georgia. He suffered a traumatic brain injury in October of 2007, while he was a senior at Roswell High School. After a stay at the Shepherd Center, he was blessed to go on to Oglethorpe University to receive his bachelor's degree in playwriting. From there, he went to Boston University to receive his M.F.A in Playwriting, and then, he went on to the University of Louisville to receive a master's degree in teaching. He is now a Limited-term Assistant Professor of English at Kennesaw State University. He loves his job, sharing his story with his students, and hoping to encourage and inspire them on to live their lives to the fullest.

The Far Reaches of Traumatic Brain Injury and Grief

By Norma Myers

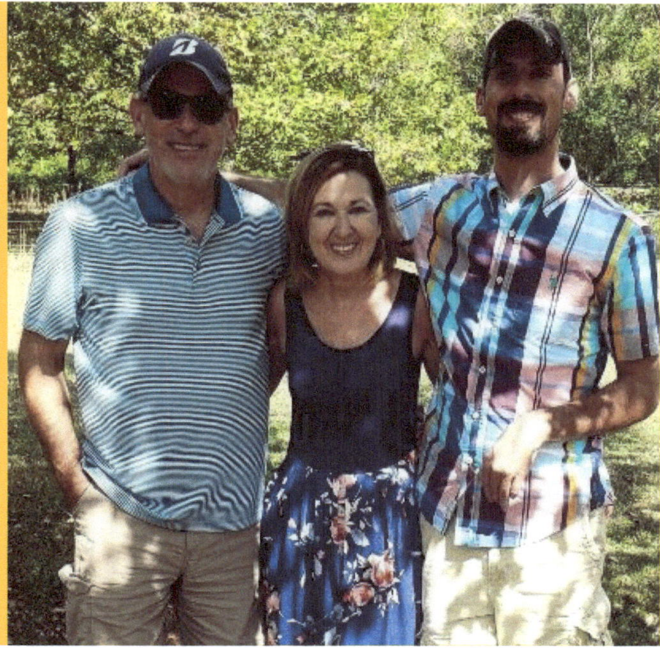

While my thoughts should have been carefree during our summer vacation at our favorite North Carolina beach, each day as I took in the vastness of the ocean, I was reminded of the far reaches of traumatic brain injury (TBI) and grief.

Our carefree days came to an end on August 13, 2012 when our sons, Aaron and Steven, were involved in a fatal car accident — an accident that took Aaron away from us and left Steven with a severe TBI. Upon receiving the horrific news of the fatal accident, we had no idea at the time how double trauma would impact the world around us. Not only would we forever grieve the earthly separation from Aaron, but we would be faced with navigating the foreign soil of TBI and the many layers entangled within this life-changing, invisible disease. We learned very quickly that instead of fearing words such as "TBI," "epilepsy," "PTSD," and "complicated grief" (just to scratch the surface), we had to become educated advocates.

> "Seven years later, we still find ourselves trying to fill in gaps of time where dismal fog set in, leaving us with amnesia."

When speaking of "far reaches," there's not enough space to cover all the territory touched by our journey! It's not just about us; it's about our family, friends, employers, and community. At some level, they also felt our gut-wrenching blow! They rallied around us, allowing us to draw strength from their hopefulness, which we needed during our darkest of days when we felt anything but hopeful.

Once the initial shock started wearing off, we desperately wanted and needed to piece those first minutes, hours, and days back together. Seven years later, we still find ourselves trying to fill in gaps of time where dismal fog set in, leaving us with amnesia. We were truly operating on auto-pilot, doing what needed to be done to be there for Steven and somehow managing to plan Aaron's life celebration, hoping and praying that we honored our firstborn son in the beautiful way that he so deserved.

"Far reaches" also means letting go of pride, the same pride that in the past would have caused us to say no to help. We're beyond thankful for every individual, healthcare provider, and organization that was there to say, "Yes, we will help!" Many remain in our lives today, cheering us on!

Some of the unpleasant "far reaches" include helping Steven navigate the chaos of Social Security, insurance denials, the never-ending hospital bills, not to mention encounters with people that don't understand that it's okay to ask about Steven's deficits instead of avoiding or reacting as if TBI is contagious! Those are a few examples of the uglies you don't want your 29-year-old son subjected to, ever! Being a Mama Bear that has been by her son's side as he fought his way back to life, it's natural to want to protect Steven from anything painful. But, oh, how well I have learned … that's just not possible. So each time I witness Steven's patience and grace as he handles heavy burdens at his young age, my ears hear the loud, melodious message of hope … Steven's got this!

I never imagined facing a crisis of this magnitude, one that has changed me physically, emotionally, and spiritually. Trauma is two-sided. While I don't ignore the painful side (as I endure the side effects of trauma each day), I prefer to focus on the positives. I love more deeply. I embrace hope like never before. I hug tighter. I don't rush, which helps me appreciate the here and now. I hurt for those that hurt. I count every blessing. And I'm not ashamed of my tears.

As parents, it's only natural to think about your child's future. We find ourselves in "what if" conversation about Aaron on a regular basis. Would Aaron be married? Would we be grandparents? Our conversations are different regarding Steven. Our hearts hurt knowing Steven has physical and emotional pain that he deals with each day, without complaint. Due to Steven's TBI, he had no idea until weeks following the accident that his brother, his best friend, didn't survive. Steven didn't get to be a part of Aaron's life celebration. Whether that's a blessing or a curse, it's still a part of Steven's reality. Our reality. Those are the kind of "far reaches" of TBI and grief that feel like a vise-grip around my heart.

Professionals say there are seven stages of grief. I agree with the written seven. But trust me. There are so many more, especially regarding complicated grief. Until I became a mother that heard the words, "your son didn't survive," I thought all grief was complicated, but the most complicated of all is truly child loss.

On my most challenging days, I purposely remember the far reaches of Aaron's love, his passion for the great outdoors, his smile and compassion for everyone. Those treasures, coupled with Steven's sheer determination to continue honoring his promise to Aaron to never give up are the memories and moments, past and present, that keep me showing up to be the wife that Carlan needs, be the mother that keeps Aaron's beautiful memory alive, be Steven's faithful cheerleader, and be there for our family, friends, and community, like they are always there for us.

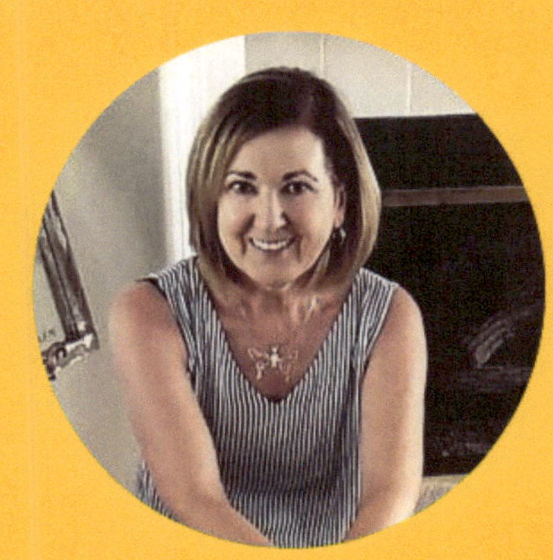

Meet Norma Myers

Norma and her husband Carlan spend much of their time supporting their son Steven as he continues on his road to recovery after sustaining a Traumatic Brain Injury in 2012. Carlan faithfully supports his family while working full-time in his demanding Human Resources career. The Myers family are advocates for those recovering from Traumatic Brain Injury and for those that have also experienced child loss.

"Have enough courage to trust love one more time and always one more time."

— *Maya Angelou*

Our Creativity is Waiting to Re-Emerge

By Judith Johnston

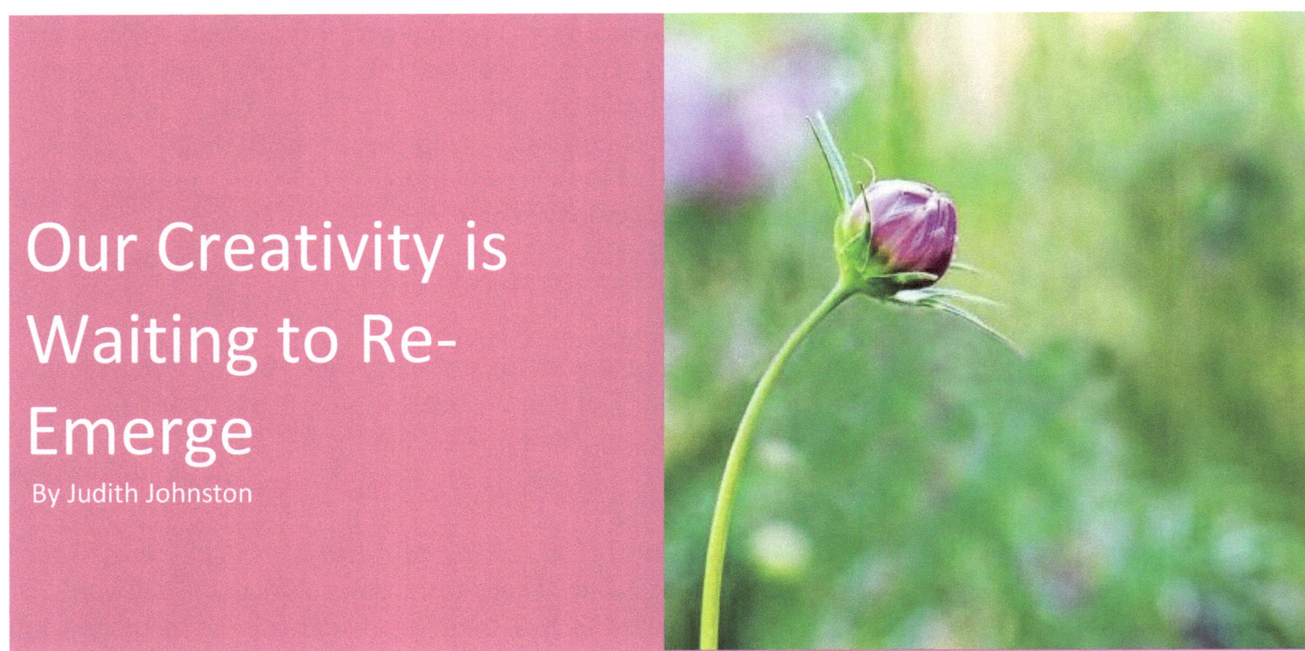

Think about those creative activities or interests that you liked to pursue during your childhood. Was it drawing or painting, playing an instrument or singing, writing short stories, building model ships or planes, anything that held you captive as you created something new or continued to build onto an interest or avocation you truly enjoyed doing?

In my pre-ABI life's story, I grew up as the eldest of nine children, went to university, entered the work force and became an Employee Benefits Consultant. I married much later in life and as a result of my husband's interests, I learned to like basketball which, in turn, led us to becoming the active, committed and loving guardians of a teenaged boy who continues to make us proud in so many ways.

> "Then, in an instant, my life changed. Almost six years ago I suffered a catastrophic ABI as a result of a car accident."

All of this was happening as I tried my best to provide emotional and personal support to others that needed me to be there for them. Then, in an instant, my life changed. Almost six years ago I suffered a catastrophic ABI as a result of a car accident. It has been a life of ups and downs, trials and tribulations, backsliding and achievements.

There is no question that this life challenge has slowed me down, but I am learning how not to allow it to become a permanent obstacle to my continued growth as a productive human being, as I move forward on this unexpected journey. It is my belief that prior to our being impacted by an acquired brain injury we are all, in some way, affected by the proverbial treadmill of the "daily grind." Over time those seemingly routine activities quickly turned into an avalanche of unmitigated responsibilities.

We are left with little or no personal time for engaging in those past creative pursuits. Eerily, I found I had become unaware of how these pre-ABI life responsibilities took away my creative "ME" time. The reality is that, now, as we learn to again breathe, putting one foot in front of the other and begin to move forward with our lives, we find those past life responsibilities had succeeded in pulling us away from engaging in long ago life fulfilling and socially enriching activities. In this journey of coming to terms with my brain injury, I am finding my creative "ME" side once again. This took time, almost three years from the day of my car accident.

It took the cajoling, suggestions and patience of those around me to allow me to find my way back to those things I did in my youth. It also took learning about how to become mindful and grounded with the help of meditation so that I could find myself once again. Because of the support of those around me I am richer in spirit for finding my way back to writing, drawing and a newly discovered passion for painting watercolors. Each activity energizes me, making me feel a personal sense of fulfilment and self-accomplishment.

One of the unexpected benefits to finding my way back to art as a hobby is that I am less critical of the process and of how my watercolors turn out. They are truly works in progress just as I am. Even though my art teacher finds she has to repeat examples of techniques we learned in previous classes, I am okay with that. When I was in high school, I always felt pressured to be the best I could be and then some.

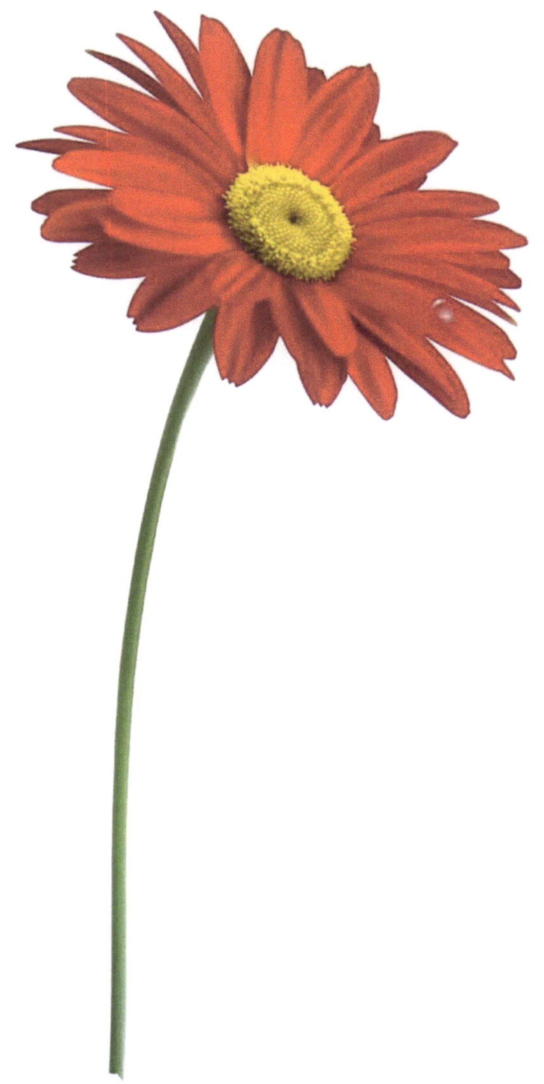

"In this journey of coming to terms with my brain injury, I am finding my creative "ME" side once again."

I had a grandmother who was an artist, and her high expectations were not lost on me. Despite winning the Art Award in my final year, I constantly questioned my abilities and creativeness. Now, as I continue to move forward in my recovery from an ABI, I have inexplicably been able to find a new enjoyment by coming back to those creative activities I once engaged in.

For me, a benefit of having survived a brain injury is that now I am not so hard on myself when working on a painting. I have no one I need to please or impress. I can accept in myself the knowing when a piece is finished, or if it is better that I step away and begin something new. Regardless, I am able to spend just over an hour of my time by putting my singular focus and concentration into working on a watercolor.

Yes, it exhausts me, but it has become a positive cognitive form of exhaustion. Give yourself a goal. My goal is to work towards increasing the once weekly activity into a multiple weekly occurrence as a way of challenging my brain. It may be something you did before your ABI. It can be something, that until now, you haven't given much thought to trying it out.

To make a start in reactivating your creative side, how about working on a puzzle, or coloring in one of the many whimsical coloring books out there, or maybe it is putting your energy into looking at and cataloguing past and present family photos.

Even if you need someone to help you with that endeavor, the positive impact to your well-being is that you will light up when you are able to carry it through, by talking about it in a social setting, with self-pride. Find your escape back to what you enjoyed doing in your youth and allow those experiences to help you move forward. It's made a big difference in my life, and it can in yours – only if you are willing to try it!

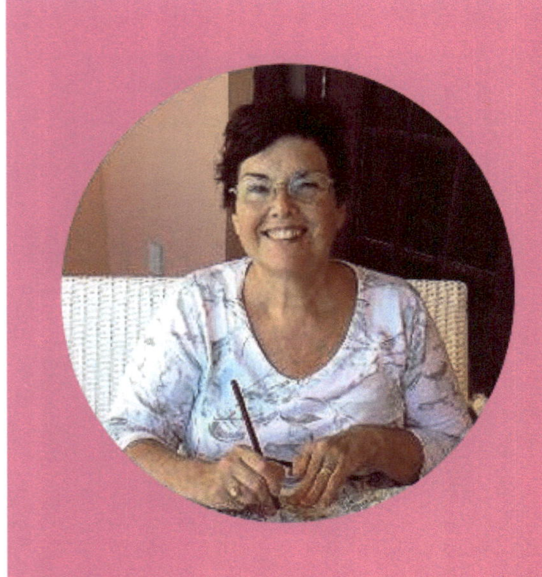

Meet Judith Johnston

In 2014, Judith Johnston, a Vice President and Employee Benefit Consultant, was on her way to see a client when, as a result of a car accident, her life changed dramatically. A passionate presenter, along with her foray into creative writing, Judith instills hope and promotes collaboration amongst survivors, caregivers and professionals. In this role she empowers us all as we each make this journey. Her blog is entitled "My Journey with ABI" and can be found at www.abimyjourney.com

Living Life on Life's Terms

By James Scott

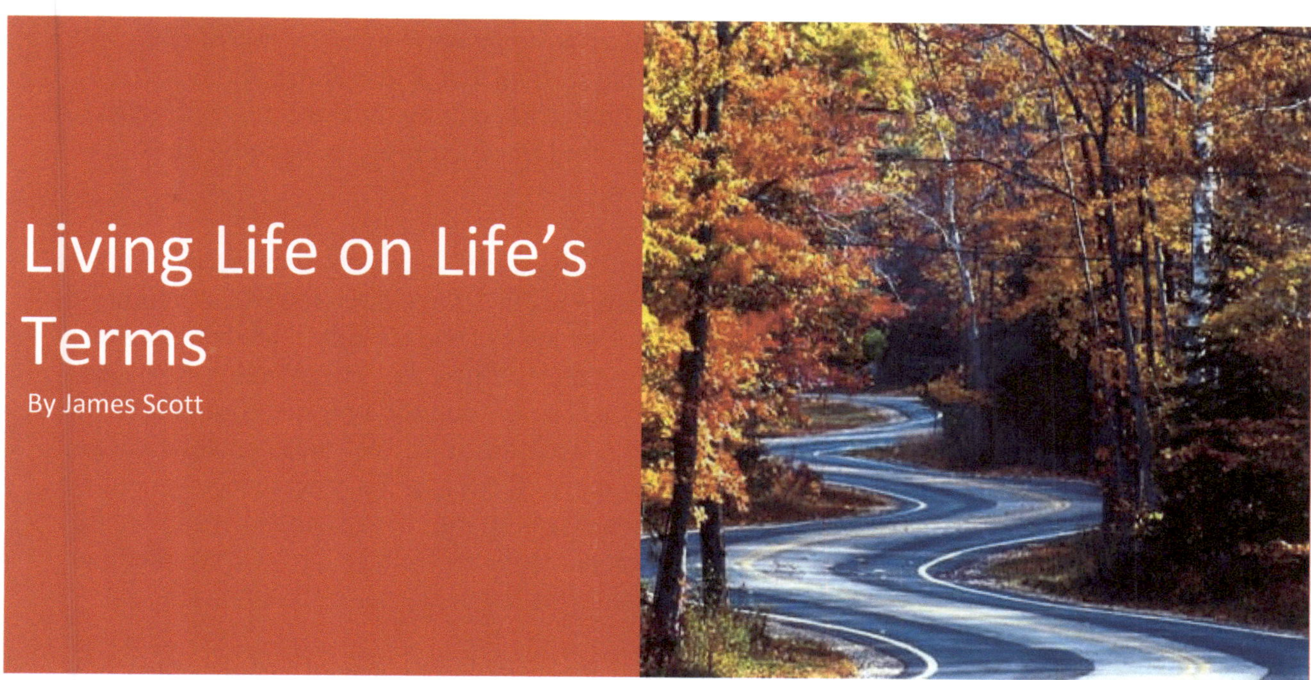

It seems that acceptance is a word that is thrown around often in recovery communities. Whether it be recovery after a brain injury, a sudden loss, or after brain injury, acceptance is nearly always one of the most important steps in an individuals' journey. Of course, I speak with the benefit of having my vision greatly enhanced by hindsight. It's not as though after I woke up a hemiplegic, my cognition and emotion regulation greatly impaired, to the mantra, *"Acceptance is the springboard to recovery!"*

In fact, it was over a year until I began to grasp that, although blessed with the chance to live and see recovery gains in the aftermath of a severe injury, there wouldn't be a morning that saw the old, pre-injury Jim rise again to conquer the world. And while I certainly wouldn't advise complete denial, just putting one foot in front of the other and working hard without deep reflection has served me well.

> "This slow trickle of understanding and truth about my brain injury never left me in a place of complete hopelessness or giving up."

This slow trickle of understanding and truth about my brain injury never left me in a place of complete hopelessness or giving up. I can only attribute this to the tremendous love and support of my family and social circle. For this seemingly fortunate naivete of the challenges of recovery from the permanence of brain injury, I am grateful as well as amazed at the way a lack of knowledge and inability to grasp reality served as a great protector to me. Like most words in our fickle English language, I have nowhere near a mastery of, acceptance has many meanings. While most of these definitions contain the implication of defeat or swallowing a bitter pill, personally the one I like best describes acceptance as "a willingness to tolerate a difficult situation." I love this particular entry under acceptance in the dictionary for two primary reasons: It is a stated ideal of a desired mindset with which to approach a situation, and as with most ideals, perfection is just a target. In fact, when speaking of the "willingness to tolerate" we're really talking about a future moment without any demand or expectation. The fact is that though in the actual moment we might be distressed and rageful with resistance, in opening the door to a willingness for tolerating our difficulty, we move towards that ideal. I find much comfort in avoiding viewing acceptance through black or white and success or fail lenses.

Acceptance was not something that has ever come naturally to me. I suppose that growing up in a loving family shielded me from some of the disappointments that force the issue when it comes to acquiring the "acceptance skill." Then again, perhaps I've always had a faulty understanding of acceptance as an action that bears little resemblance to the definition that I now find most fitting. Whether because of societal influences of masculinity as being a John Wayne-like figure who molds situations with sheer will, or it's just my nature, but throwing the adjective "unacceptable" on a circumstance always seemed a bit triumphant. For whatever the reason may be, it seems that I've always equated acceptance to condoning a result, and perhaps worse for this stubborn New Englander, giving up hope for better or any improvement. With this mindset, it's no wonder that becoming comfortable with my new life after brain injury has been a long, difficult process.

When I say this, please understand that in no way am I trying to paint a dismal picture of my life today, nor am I looking for sympathy. In fact, my life is great! I have a solid support network of family and friends along with an amazing woman with two young boys. Letting me be a part of their life has been an absolute blessing. As I write this today, I can't help but ask myself how I got so lucky as to deserve this incredible outcome. This leads me to another important point about acceptance - it's not just the difficult situations or losses that can be a challenge to accept.

It can be easy for me to put the blame for my self-recriminating thoughts and almost constant feelings of unworthiness on the cause of my car crash and TBI being entirely my fault from driving drunk. In fact, the feelings of guilt and self-loathing have nearly been unbearable. As counterintuitive as it may sound, I've really had to learn to accept the good, and found it just as difficult as accepting loss and disappointment. The cognitive dissonance surrounding a joyous life after a horrible mistake leads me fighting the urge to self-sabotage. As more is revealed to me each day, it is becoming apparent that only when I learn to embrace each moment as it comes, will I truly be living a life of true and meaningful acceptance.

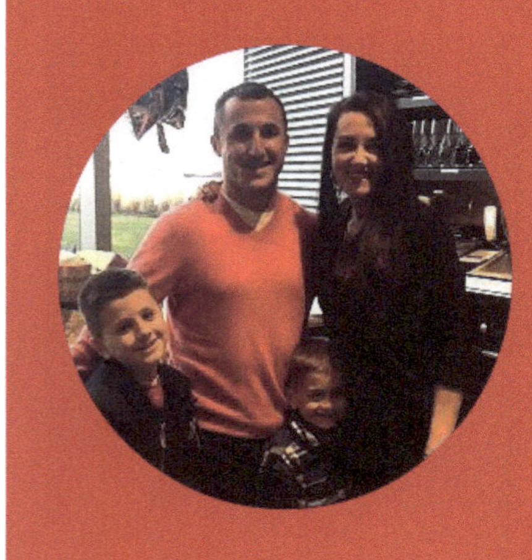

Meet James Scott

After growing up in Atkinson, NH and then graduating from the University of Tampa, Jim sustained a TBI in a motor vehicle crash in 2006. Recognizing the cautionary value in his personal story, as his crash was caused by impaired driving, Jim first began speaking to students with KC's Community Education program. In order to increase the number of people reached, Jim has also worked with Northeast Rehabilitation Hospital's Think First National Injury Prevention Foundation. In 2012, Jim published a memoir titled *More Than a Speed Bump: Life Before and After Traumatic Brain Injury.*

An Ordinary Day?

By Russ Cobleigh

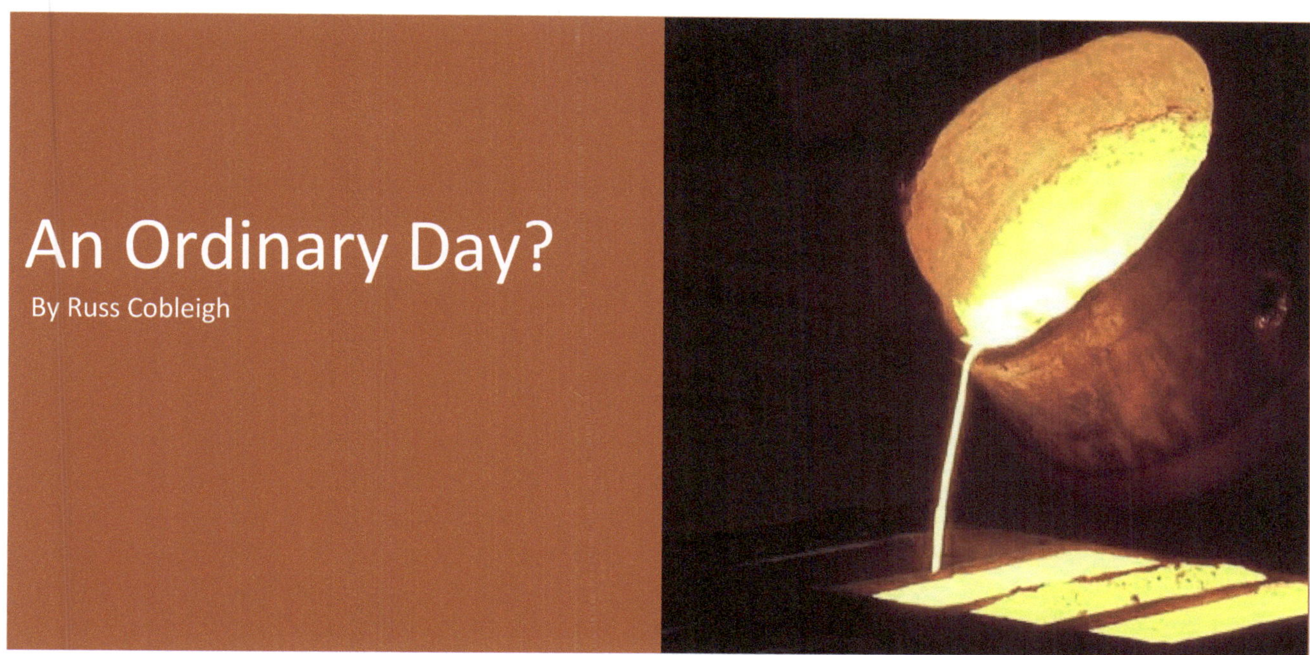

December 9, 2015 was supposed to be an ordinary day. I had recently been hired in a full-time position at a smelting factory in Bredaryd. It was not my top job choice, but a job was a job. I had just come back from breakfast and started up the press that I had been working at for a couple of months. Everything was going normal. I had my music on with earbuds, so I never knew what was coming.

I remember a bright light, and then something hitting me hard on the head and neck. I then realized that I was on the floor. I looked up and saw that the overhead lamp had come loose and hit me. It was just hanging there. I don't really remember how long I waited before someone came and helped me up and took me into the floor manager's office. I was asked if I was okay, but don't remember what I said. I was told to go home and that if I did not feel better, I should call the doctor.

> "I remember a bright light, and then something hitting me hard on the head and neck. I then realized that I was on the floor."

This meant that I had to walk to the bus stop, a five-to-seven minute walk away. At that point, I then had to wait for the next bus which could have been anywhere between half an hour and an hour. Lastly, I had to take the thirty minute bus ride home. Once home, it was then suggested that someone take me to the ER, which is exactly what happened.

I got to the ER and had to wait to be shown into an exam room. I was asked a couple of questions and was told I was being sent to x-ray to check for broken bones. There was no concussion check and no CT scan. I went down and got ex-rayed and they had to wheel me back upstairs because I felt dizzy. In all, I was in and out of the hospital in under two hours, all this after a severe work accident. The next day my head and neck were hurting. I went to my local doctor and was given a vague diagnosis, two weeks sick leave and sent home. I then went to my union and gave them my doctor's note and tried to report the accident. I was told the person handling my case was on vacation and someone would contact me, and then sent home. After the two weeks was up, I went back to work, not knowing what else to do and getting no meaningful advice from anyone.

I tried to tell them the doctor spoke of Post-Concussion Syndrome. As I had no broken bones, I was told to simply go back to work, as if nothing had happened. I went back to the same press where my injury occurred. I was scared and nervous. As the next couple of weeks went by, my neck really started hurting and I went back to the doctor. I was told that I could get more sick time, but that he would have to write down in my journal that I had asked for more time. I had never been told that by a doctor before and it freaked me out, so I went back to work.

Over the next few months my neck got worse and I started feeling really weird. I would often get dizzy. Lights, sounds and smells would start bothering me and I started forgetting things. I was pretty much ignored at work. In May I went back to the doctors and asked for a new doctor. My new doctor said that I had been going through whiplash and had sustained a concussion. He gave me additional sick leave - sick leave that I am still on to this day. Six months after the accident I finally was sent to get a CT scan. The scan showed nothing, though by now it was six months after the accident. I was turned down four times to see a neurologist because they said my pacemaker was an issue. I was sent to a rehab center, which meant having to take the train to the next big town - Jönköping. I had to stay in a hotel for three days and have about six to seven hours of different group sessions. At this time things were really getting weird. Life was difficult. Being around too many people freaked me out and being alone in the hotel was so lonely.

One day at the hospital we were in the large dining hall and I swear I could hear everybody. It scared me so badly that I actually had to leave. I did this rehab for a couple of weeks, but I just could not handle all the train travel, hotel, and group sessions. It was just too much for me. No one here was talking to me about sensory overload, or brain fog or the tinnitus that was and is slowly driving me mad. I have to stop now my eyes are tired, my ears are ringing, and my neck is hurting.

As of today, I still have received no compensation for my work accident. My life is difficult, and I hope that it will get better. But most of all, I hope that my story will help someone.

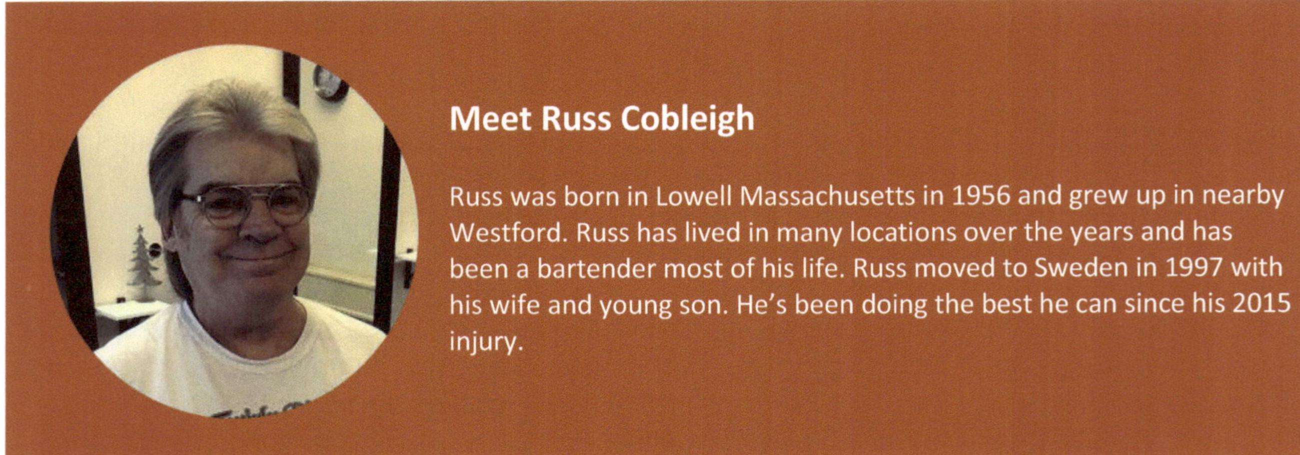

Meet Russ Cobleigh

Russ was born in Lowell Massachusetts in 1956 and grew up in nearby Westford. Russ has lived in many locations over the years and has been a bartender most of his life. Russ moved to Sweden in 1997 with his wife and young son. He's been doing the best he can since his 2015 injury.

Finding Hope

By Dr. Edward King

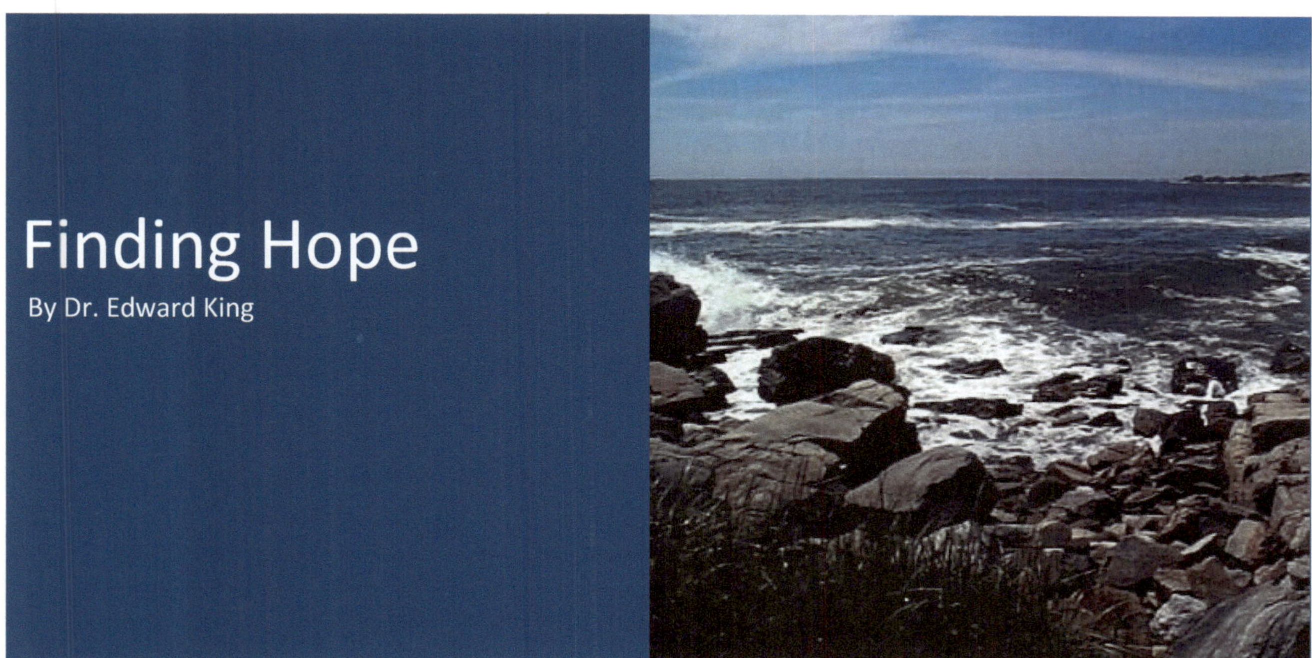

Not long following my stroke of 2003, I was of the opinion that my chances for success in any of my remaining physician skills; lay somewhere between little to none. The several months immediately post stroke my therapy took place at The Lahey Clinic in Burlington, Massachusetts. Most of my therapy venues post stroke have been under the supervision of occupational therapists at Portsmouth Hospital's Neuro Day Rehab Center for Rehabilitation. One of the OT's mantras was to focus upon what you can do, as opposed to what you cannot.

In retrospect, any successes I have experienced post-stroke have been a direct consequence of some pre-existing skill, or skills, I previously had. Pre stroke, one of my core competencies lay in the knowledge of how to make sailboats go fast; both upwind, and downwind. For eight summers, I had taught sailboat racing to teenagers during medical school and college. This took place at Indian Harbor Yacht Club in Greenwich, Connecticut on Long Island Sound from 1964 to 1972.

> "One of the Occupational Therapist's mantras was to focus upon what you CAN do, as opposed to what you cannot do."

My first post stroke sailing appearance was at Piers Park, well prior to going to the United States Sailing Men's Championships. Those skills translated into two podium appearances in the United States Sailing National Men's Disabled Sailing Regattas in 2011 and 2013. Both of these podium appearances were accompanied by fellow Krempels Center member, fellow crewmate, Jim Scott III. It was through my connections to Northeast Passage, that I first learned of an adaptive sailing facility in Boston, Massachusetts at Harbor Piers Park.

At the time it was run by a lady named Maureen McKinnon-Tucker. She had won an adaptive sailing Olympic gold medal in the recent Paralympics in Beijing, China. For one of my best Father's Days ever, my older son, Robbie, treated his Mom and me to a Boston Harbor sailing excursion, one which I'll never forget!

UNH's Northeast Passage in Durham, New Hampshire offers graduate degrees in the discipline of Therapeutic Recreation. They are very involved in helping disabled folks return to adaptive sports. They are also closely associated with Krempels Center for Brain Injury Survivors in Portsmouth, New Hampshire, which I attend three days a week. Northeast Passage brought adaptive cycling to Krempels Center. I fell in love with an adaptive recumbent three wheeler bike called, "The Green Speed." I rode one of them in two "Tours de Cure" on the New Hampshire seacoast. Not long afterwards my family acquired one of them for my very own. I'm pleased to ride it in the annual King Challenge around Columbus Day in autumn.

The King Challenge has become one of the true joys of my life. Our entire family joins in. Each year sees a reunion of like-minded friends of Krempels Center. This takes place on the campus of the Timberland Company world headquarters in Stratham, New Hampshire. Each year, over three hundred cyclists raise over $100,000. All of which goes to support Krempels Center for brain injury survivors.

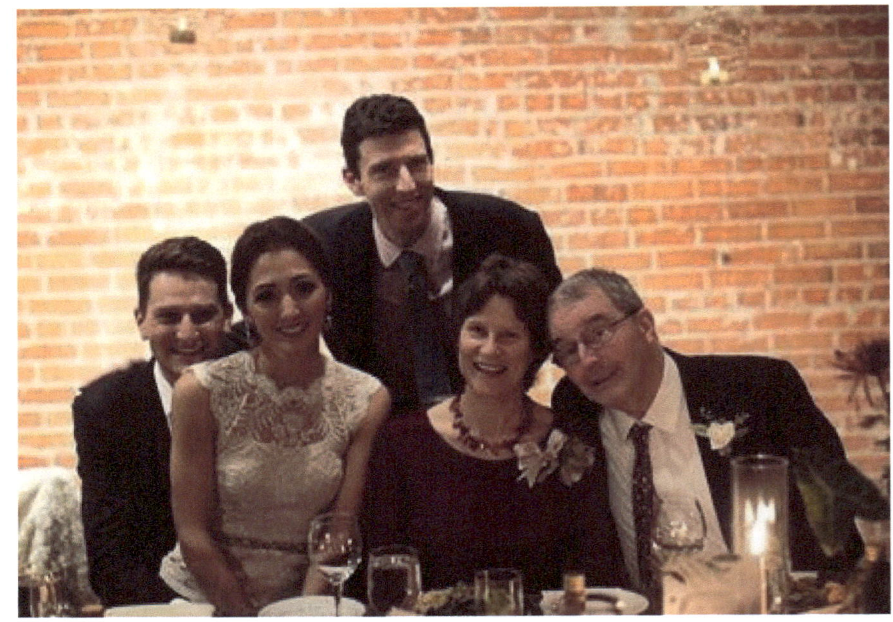

Adaptive skiing was my next sport. Something called motor memory has played an important role in both my sailing, and skiing successes. By that, I mean that it is second nature to me. How to steer a sailboat, or a bicycle, or even a pair of skis, no matter the condition that confronts me. Whether I'm cycling, sailing, or even downhill skiing!

Four years of youth piano lessons, the ability to read music, and some choir singing experiences were other preexisting skills of mine. Which in turn, post stroke, led me to join my Exeter, New Hampshire church choir, and subsequent singing performances with The Rockingham County's Men's Choral Societies'. With them I had performances singing "The Navy Hymn," at two memorial services, for a surgical colleague's wife, on one given day. They were held in both Exeter and Stratham, New Hampshire Congregational Church's memorial services.

Creative writing, in the genre of creative nonfiction, has become another passion of mine. This is the genre of memoir writing. Sometime after my 2003 stroke, I told my spouse Margie that I should either be writing a memoir or keeping a journal to record many of the ironic happenings of my new life post stroke. Soon afterwards, Margie called my attention to a memoir writers group meeting at the Exeter Public Library in New Hampshire. That first session was given by an instructor named, Nancy Eichhorn. She had taught memoir writing to students from elementary grade levels, to graduate students. Her thesis, was that the creative juices of a writer's mind, can be aided by a prompt. This prompt can be as simple as a few words of a poem, or a song.

Since then, many of us Writers of the Round Table, have assembled every Tuesday morning. As Writers of the Round Table, we have published four volumes, each titled, "Prompted to Write." As a member, I have been either the author, or coauthor of these four volumes.

Here at Krempels Center, a day program in New Hampshire for those affected by brain injury, after picking a random prompt, we write for twenty minutes before dropping our pens, to read aloud to one another. Only constructive criticism is permitted. One lesson from this writing exercise lies in the fact that most of us, have some level of talent in certain skills, artistic, athletic, or even intellectual. To capitalize on those skills has been a wonderful experience. For some of us, it has restored more meaning and a sense of true fulfillment to our lives.

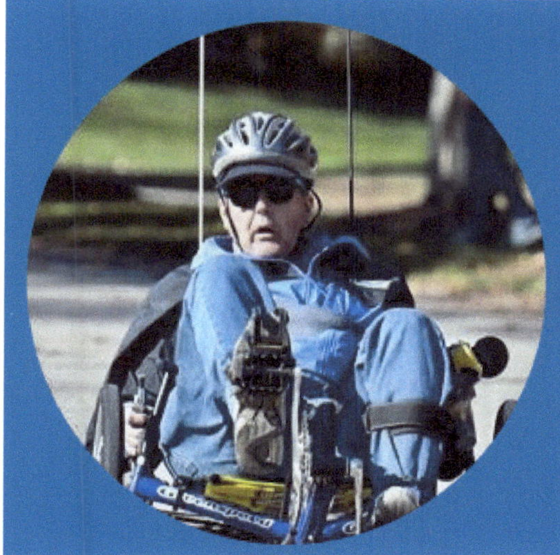

Meet Dr. Edward King

Dr. Edward W. King is a happily retired general orthopedic surgeon. He retired after surviving a massive stroke that left him as a left hemiplegic. He has been married 48 years to Margaret, the mother of the two King brothers, Robbie and Teddy. He is a lifelong sailor and enjoys painting. Ted is an expert in sailing, having raced nineteen across the North Atlantic Gulf Stream to Bermuda. Ted also is an active participant at Krempels Center in Portsmouth, New Hampshire.

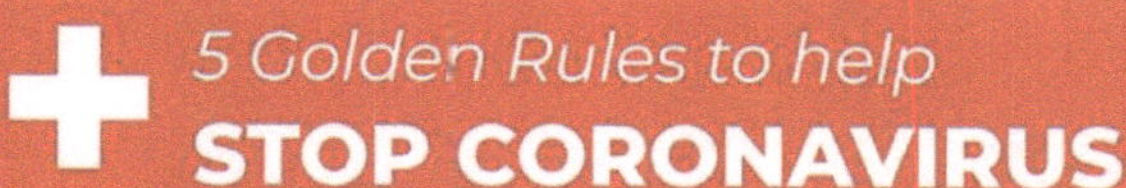

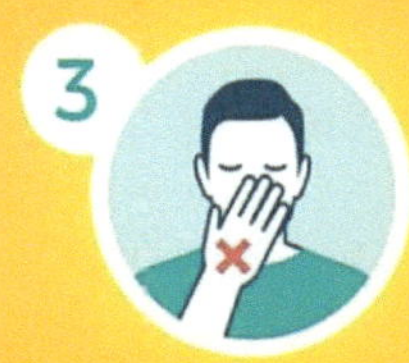

The POWER Of Support Groups

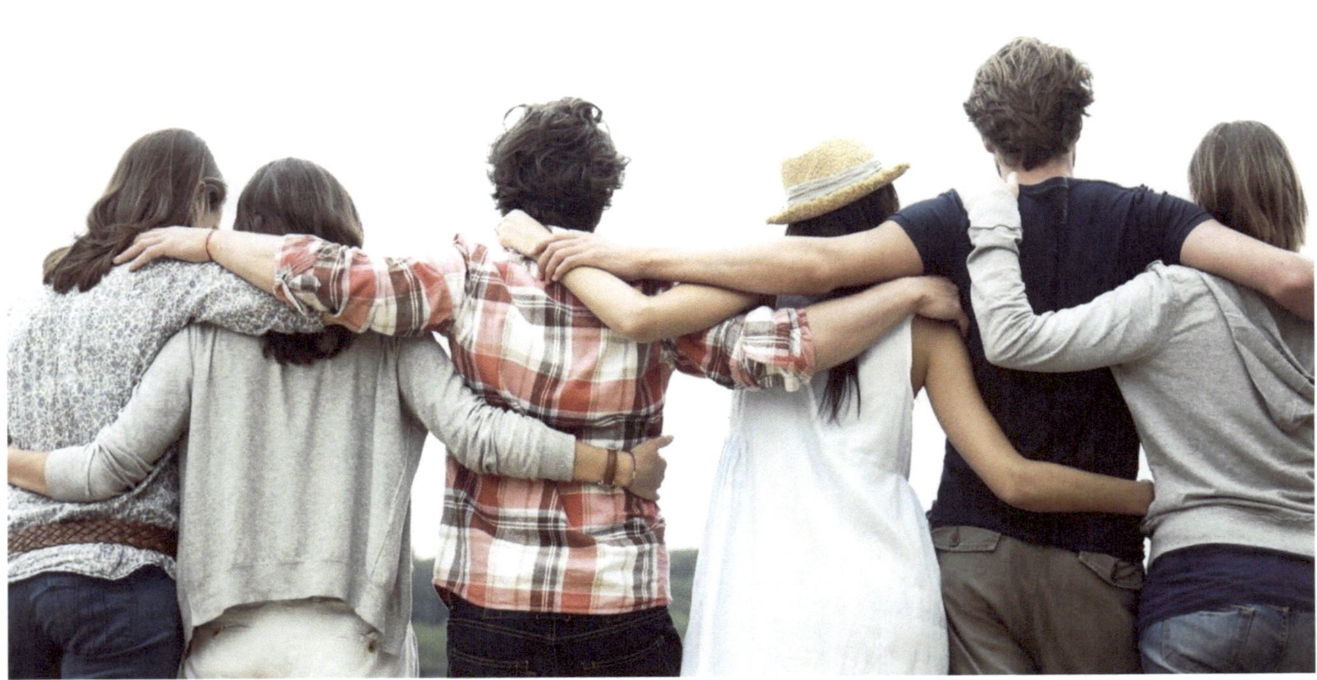

A Lighthouse in the Night

By Rachel Dombeck

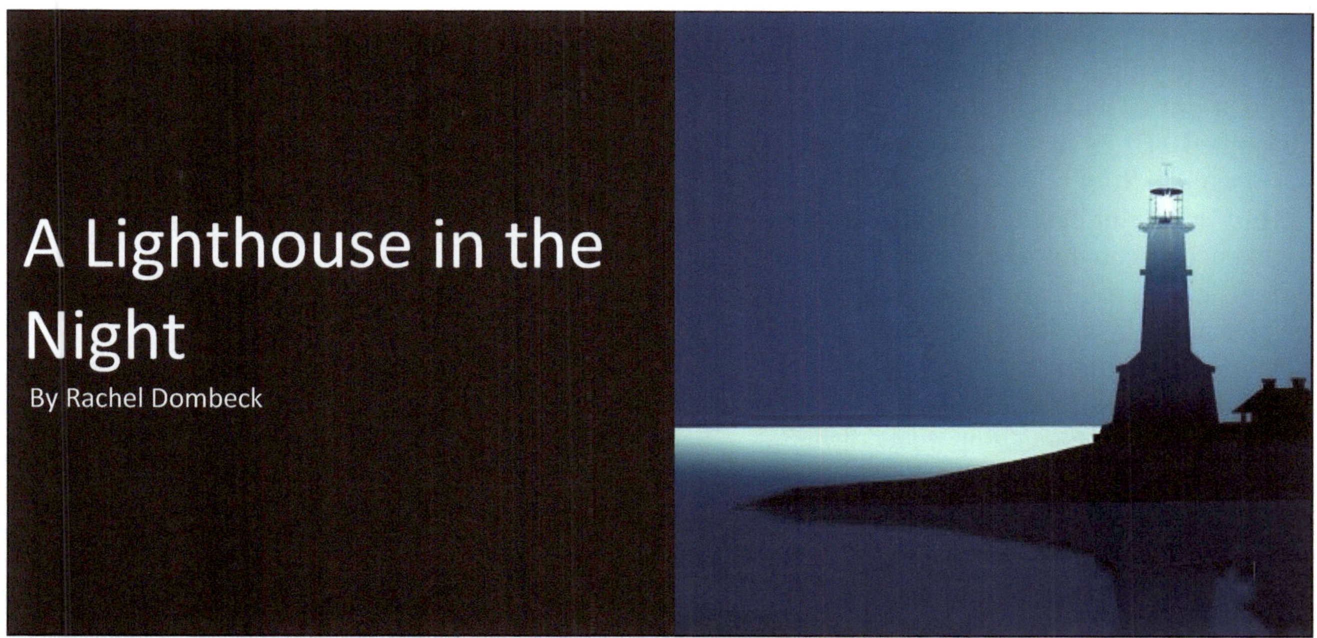

When I saw the opportunity to write and share about support groups, I was very excited and jumped at the chance to speak of the huge benefit they can have in your recovery.

Where to start? There is so much I could say, and my heart is overflowing with gratitude, love, and appreciation for the healing my support groups have brought me. We are not created to do this life alone, and even more so if we are in a turbulent time. No one is prepared for a traumatic brain injury, or any kind of brain injury. No one is given a handbook and told the ABC's of how to recover and rebuild their life. No one is held by the hand and walked through all the confusing parts of recovery that include a list longer than I could fit into this article.

> "No one is prepared for a traumatic brain injury, or any kind of brain injury. No one is given a handbook and told the ABC's of how to recover and rebuild their life."

And so, when you emerge from that realization that you are forever changed, and you are different, and you don't know yourself let alone have people that know you anymore, where do you turn? Who do you go to in the dark foggy mist of brain injury recovery?

And that is where support groups come in. They are like a lighthouse in the black, dark, cold night of TBI. I found mine through the Facebook group run by David Grant, and this magazine right here, so it is only fitting I would write and share about it here as well! I knew I needed help, I knew something was definitely not okay, and I could not seem to just "get it together and push through" as I had always done before in my life.

It was simple – thank God for the day and age we live in with technology and social media. All of that is a HUGE help and support. I simply searched TBI groups on Facebook and this one popped up. After a few weeks of following the group and being fed with helpful information and encouragement where I finally didn't feel alone, crazy, or like I was losing my mind, I saw a post about a support group, but it was in another state. I thought that is what I needed and there had to be one in my area. After looking through the list, contacting a few different groups via email and phone, I walked into a church a few weeks later where the group was held, by myself, not knowing anyone, and introduced myself.

If you read that sentence right, you get how hard that was. How big of a step that was right there. I don't pretend that starting to visit support groups and finding the right one for you will be easy. Remember, this is the brain injury journey where nothing is easy. but it is worth it a hundred times over. And let me tell you, within minutes, I felt like I wasn't alone. I felt at home with these people, I didn't have to explain myself, I didn't have to be anything but just me, and I just let my guard down because they got it.

That was over three years ago. I still attend regularly. I cannot say enough about this group and what they have meant to me in my journey. I have shown up on good days and bad days. I have shown up and shared and other days I had no words, so I just sat and listened. I have shown up mad about my life and my situation, and I have shown up grateful and happy about some good new things happening in my life. I have shown up wanting to quit, and I have shown up not knowing how to keep going on this TBI journey.

The point is, *I kept showing up*. They are a family to me. It is a safe place, it is a place where I can go and just be me, whoever that is as I figured it out along the way.

There is healing in community. There is healing in reaching out to others. By being part of a support group it's not just about you, it's about others too. Their pain, their suffering, their joys and accomplishments. You will meet those who are worse off than you, and those who have overcome what you are facing right now. So together, everyone is stronger and better because of each one in the group. There is simply no way to put into words the power of a support group. It is a place of synergy. You show up and you give, and you receive, and through that you are stronger to go out and face the next day in your journey.

I cannot encourage you enough to find a group and plug in. I have visited several, and while I make one my regular place to be a part of, I am still friends with a girl I met at a group I went to only once. We still text, I visit her from time to time and she is a huge blessing to me. I have

> "Research shows that when we reach out to others in a supportive way, we increase our own healing by a factor of 63 percent. We are designed to support each other!"
> ~Dr Caroline Leaf; Think, Learn, Succeed.

started to attend another local group recently, and feel it is time to enlarge my space of support by adding that to my schedule.

As I sat in the meeting this week, I was reminded once again how much we need each other. As a person who enjoys doing things on my own, who is naturally internally motivated, it would be easy for me to say I can do this on my own. But that is simply not true, not healthy, and not how God created us. We are created and designed for community, brain injury or not. And how much more do we require a community when we are facing a life-long condition that we must learn how to live with and navigate the best we can.

Support group and online community are huge. Please open yourself up to one and I promise that you won't regret it.

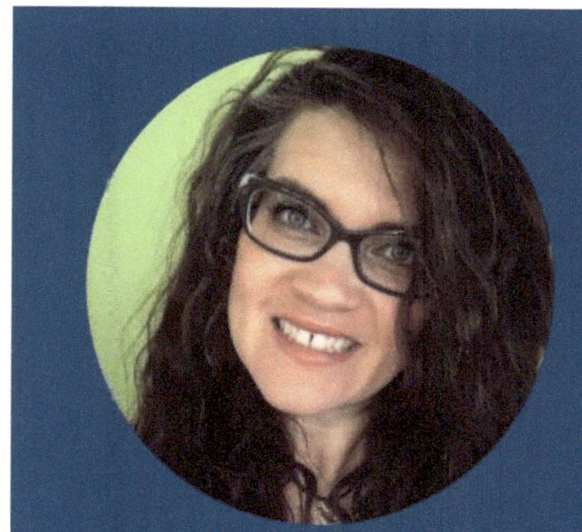

Meet Rachel Dombeck

Rachel is passionate about inspiring and empowering others in their journey while spreading awareness for brain injury and how to live a healthier life in all areas. She is learning to rebuild her life every day and finding peace in accepting the past, embracing the present and starting to dream again for the future, trusting God for the unknown.

Taking a Toll

By Ralph Poland

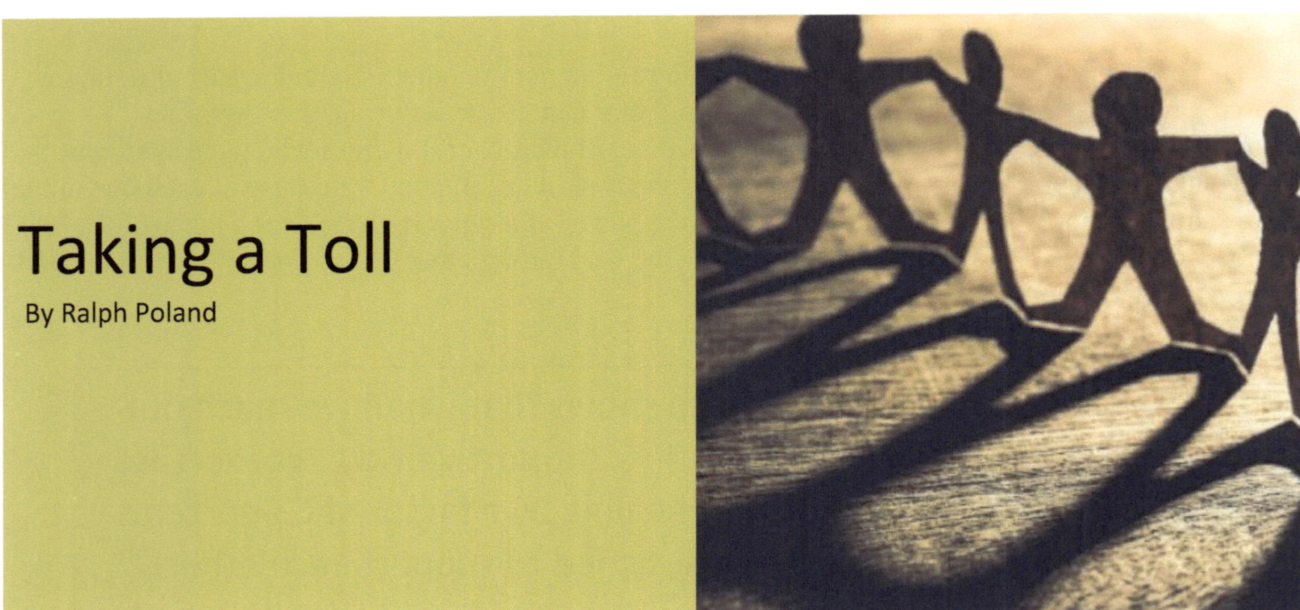

Because brain injury takes a toll on family members to whom finds themselves suddenly thrust into the world of brain injury, this can cause many of them to experience a since of being overwhelmed themselves. That is why Lewiston's brain injury support group welcomes family members of their brain injured survivor,. Whether it is a brother, sister, parent or a significant other – all are welcome to our support group. You don't even need to be accompanied by your survivor in order to attend.

Sometimes the survivor is still in the hospital. Sometimes they are in a 24/7 skilled nursing rehab facility, and there are times that he or she is not ready to attend the group yet. Family members, as well as many of the survivors in attendance, are aware that you've suddenly found yourself in a situation that can be best compared to putting a blindfold on, then trying to walk your dog.

You think you are aware of what the dog needs, but you can't even see the dog's face, let alone what is going through its mind. As the dog darts out into unexpected directions, you're quickly experiencing being overwhelmed yourself. And so it is for many of us within the brain injury community.

> "During the first part of the meeting, all attendees sit at the same table where they each can partake in conversation as they choose to do so. All conversations are centered around brain injury, where attendees are free to ask the group questions."

Because of this, our support group welcomes family members of a loved one who has acquired any type of brain injury, no matter how minor to severe.

During the first part of the meeting, all attendees sit at the same table where they each can partake in conversation as they choose to do so. All conversations are centered around brain injury, where attendees are free to ask the group questions. Others can then share about how they are coping regarding the questions asked. This allows new caregivers to hear directly from survivors about what strategies that works best for them.

At 7:00 PM, we break off into the two separate groups. The survivors continue as one group, while the caregivers move to another room. That way each group can speak freely, sharing among themselves, while finding support and learning new strategies that can be used by both survivors and caregivers within their own respected groups.

Also, while within each group, each has a chance to address one's own concerns within their group. This seems to be most helpful for attendees of both groups.

About the Lewiston, Maine Brain Injury Support Group

Our brain injury support group is held on the first Monday of the month from 6:00 PM to 8:00 PM at Westside Neuro Rehab, 618 Main Street in Lewiston, Maine. You can call 207-795-6110 for more information. This support group is open to survivors, caregivers, and family members. Our group is always reminded, "What is said in this room stays in this room!"

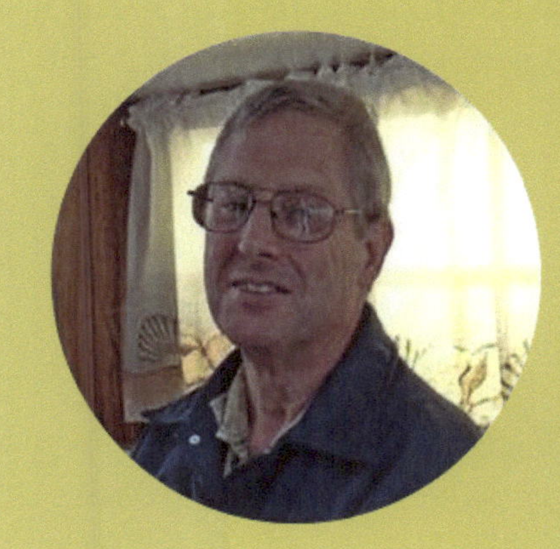

Meet Ralph Poland

Ralph's real passion is volunteering at the Rehab where he recovered. There, he shares his story with patients, offering them hope and inspiration. Ralph also serves on the BIA-MAINE Chapter, as well as on CMMC's Patient Advisory Council. He continues to offer insight from a brain injured survivor's perspective to support groups, Neuro OT students at UNE, and staff members at CMMC.

"Believe in yourself. You are braver than you think, more talented than you know, and capable of more than you imagine."

-Roy T. Bennett

What Support Groups Mean to Us

By the WINGS Brain Injury Support Group

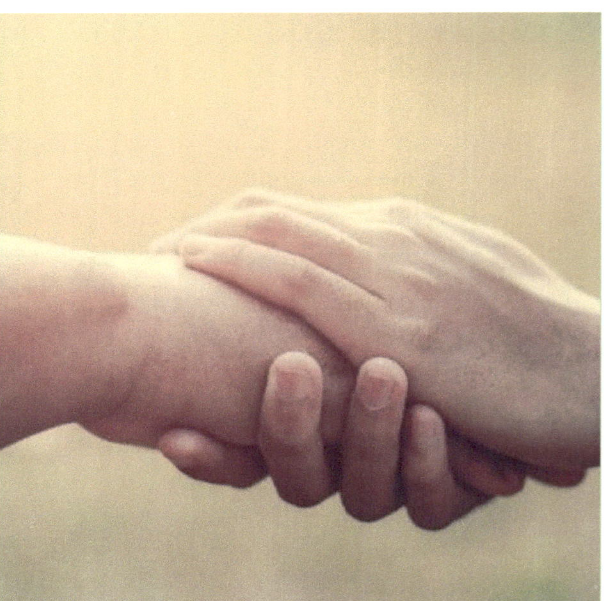

Members of the WINGS Brain Injury Support Group were asked to share what their support group meant to them. The members of this vibrant and supportive group we not shy, offering both comments as well as a vusualization of what their participation in a support group means.

"The support group has been a lifesaver, a lifeline. It's helped me to have structure when I haven't been able to be involved in things. It's given me a community and friends. It's given me access to resources and opportunities I wouldn't have found otherwise. It's been a true beacon of light through this dark time in my life." ~Zoe Dexter

"I found the support group a great place to be, a family, a group with the same issues I have, people who understand. I appreciate all the work that Brain Injury Voices puts into the support group." ~Stephanie Farrington

"Six months after my traumatic head injury, I was fortunate enough to be able to return to work. However, the transition back was very difficult. As I tried to adjust to being back, I had a lot of questions. Why was I so tired all the time? Why did I now need twelve hours of sleep and to take time off during the day? And why couldn't I remember anyone's name? I felt alone and afraid that I was the only one who experienced these issues after an injury like mine. I wondered if I would ever improve, how could I cope, who was I, now that I had lost a part of me with this injury. Even after just one session at WINGS, I knew that I had found the people that could help me answer these questions. I was reassured that I would continue to improve and that I could learn strategies to compensate for those deficits that might never go away. I now had a support group that would be there to help me address new issues as I adjusted to who I was post injury. Maybe most importantly, with their support, WINGS showed me that even though I lost some of who I was after my injury, I could also grow as I adjusted to life after my TBI." ~ Stuart Abramson

Our Support Group Means...

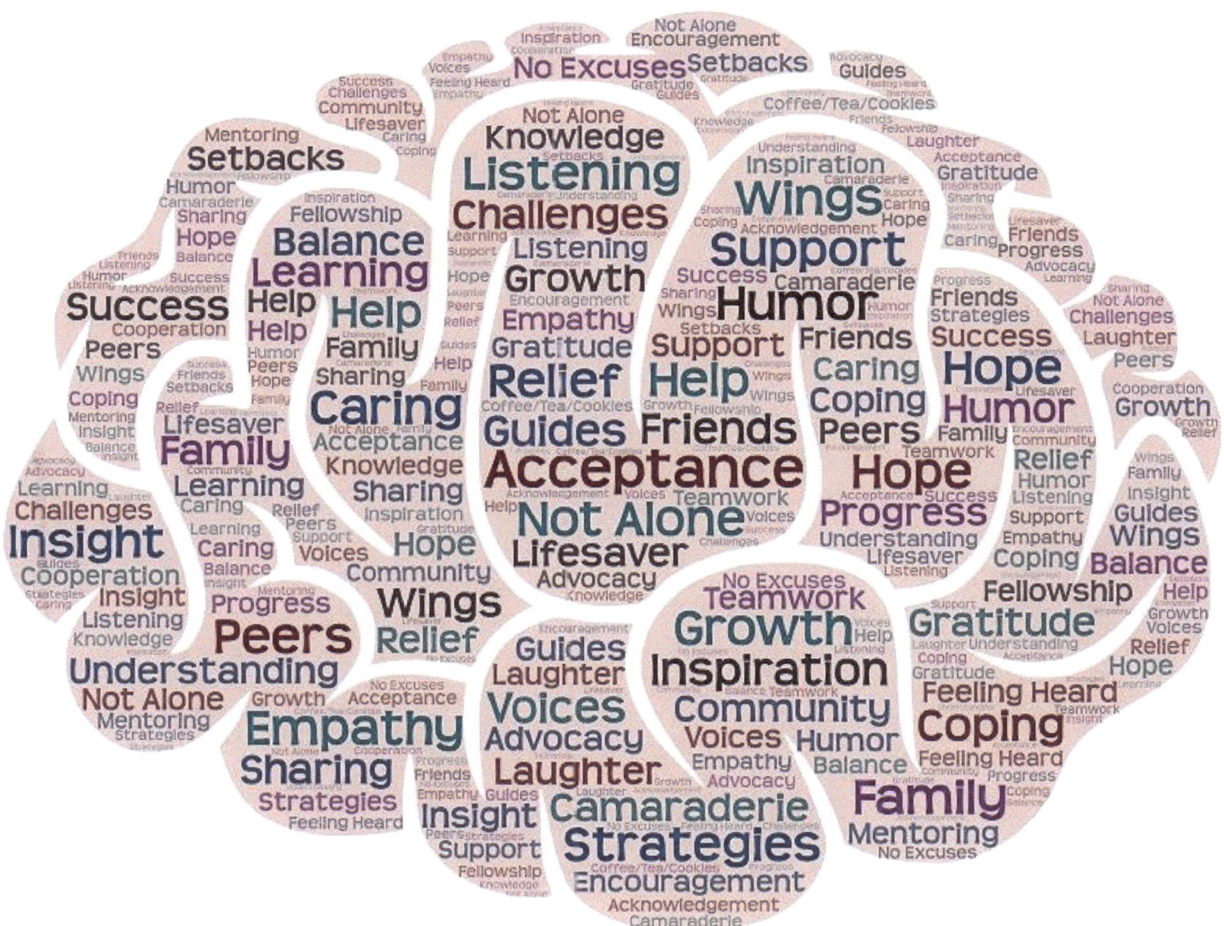

Part of Something Amazing

By Lisa Cohen Rattcliff

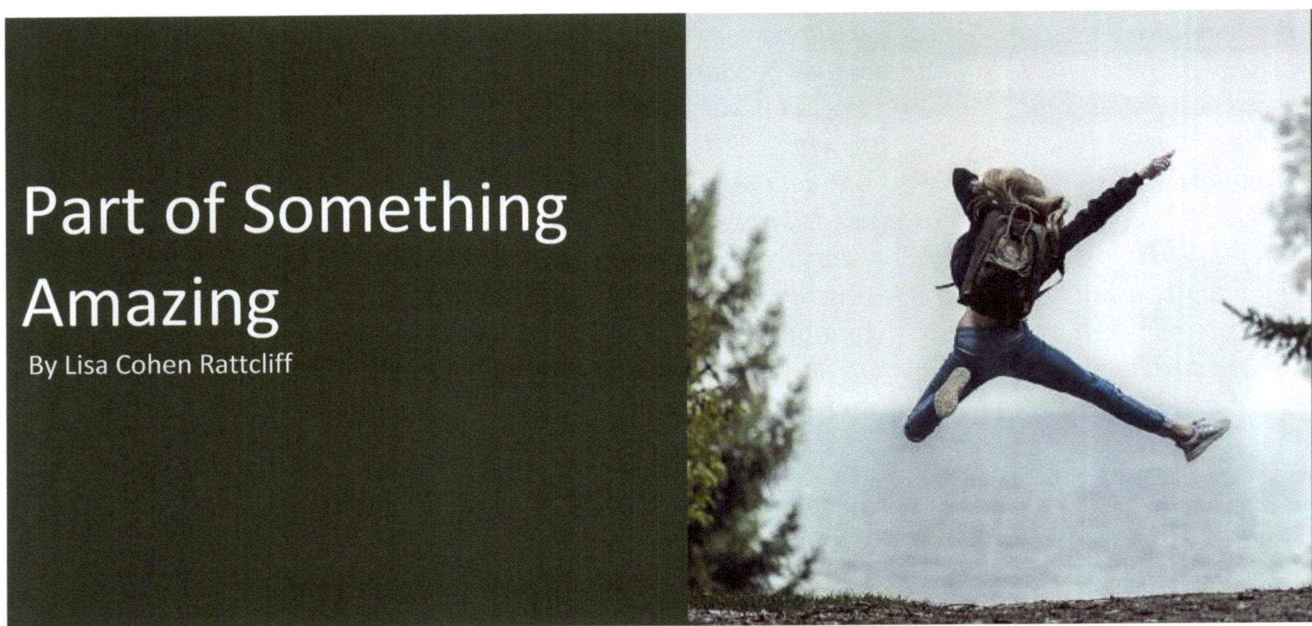

After I acquired my brain injury in 2014, I often felt I was left unequipped and too alone to pick up the remaining pieces of myself. I was suffering from the loss of my "old self," the young girl who I once was, and the life that I could never go back to. For a while I found myself lost among old friends and gatherings, I felt insecure in my inabilities and isolated at home. When my family talked about me and my situation, I sat in another room with my back against a cold sturdy sliding door, thinking they talked and talked, but they did not understand. "This is not the worst thing to ever happen to her" "Why isn't she driving yet?" "Why can't she get a job?" The voices of people often echoed in my head, they were from people I loved, but they did not have the words I needed to hear.

When doctors informed me that I should have recovered better, faster, this is as good as I will get and when doctors told me no, I thought there must be a different voice, there must be someone who understands in a way family and doctors do not. At first, I started my search online and I found great and amazing support groups that had a mass of friendly people and information.

> "I sought advice and understanding from caregivers, patients and survivors, from people who felt in pain, misunderstood and were struggling just like me."

I sought advice and understanding from caregivers, patients and survivors, from people who felt in pain, misunderstood and were struggling just like me. I loved the number of conversations, the amount of knowledge and I felt there was finally some encouragement. It was while I was in one brain injury group that I learned a very sage piece of advice. "You are your own best advocate." At the time I logged on to my online support groups I had long gaps in time where I could not see to read the text. I had experiences walking into the grocery store and then at once everything would turn blurry.

From the encouragement I gained in the online support group I learned to be more aware of my medications and recovery. One hour later, when my vision was clear, I found the boxes and containers of medications that I was on and I discovered the side effect of one medication was blurry vision. From then on out, I was looking at my recovery in a clearer light. Once I could see better, I decided I could listen better too, or at least in a different way.

Doctor after doctor contradicted themselves, saying "one day you will just wake up and all will be better" or "your eyes will never get better". From talking with other survivors, I learned about people whose eyesight improved in 5, 10, or even 20 years later. They found themselves living with improvement. I found support groups helped me to rediscover the hope that I had somehow lost along the way. True, I still had double vision and nystagmus but, I did not have to lose hope that life would remain the same way forever.

After joining online support groups, I found that I could go to a support group and meet people in my own state as well as continuing my connections with the online communities. I was a bit nervous to go in person, I was only twenty five, but I finally decided with the companionship of my mother to attend a meeting.

I am forever grateful I had the courage and support to attend my first brain injury meeting at a nearby rehabilitation center. In the beginning we went around the room and I was introduced to some truly amazing people, and I met people just like me, people with double vision, people with brain trauma, people who felt abandoned by the system, by their friends and by their doctors.

In this room passing around cookies and stories, I felt I was no longer alone. Throughout meetings I made friends, joined community events, such as the NY Brain Injury Association Walk to raise awareness and I felt part of something amazing.

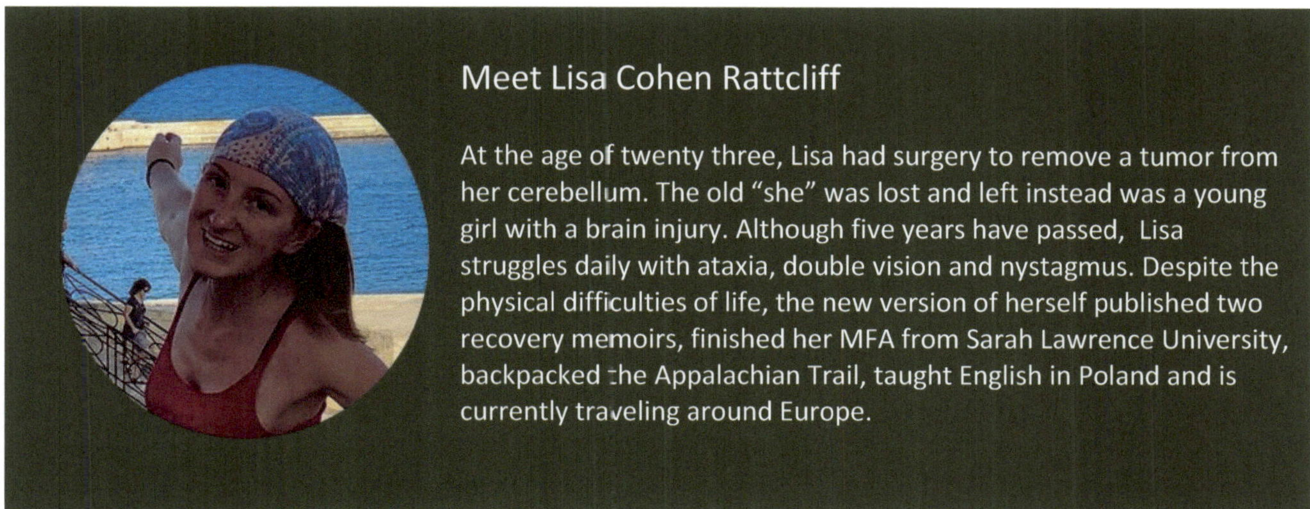

Meet Lisa Cohen Rattcliff

At the age of twenty three, Lisa had surgery to remove a tumor from her cerebellum. The old "she" was lost and left instead was a young girl with a brain injury. Although five years have passed, Lisa struggles daily with ataxia, double vision and nystagmus. Despite the physical difficulties of life, the new version of herself published two recovery memoirs, finished her MFA from Sarah Lawrence University, backpacked the Appalachian Trail, taught English in Poland and is currently traveling around Europe.

Catapulted Into Brain Injury

By Marjorie Appleby

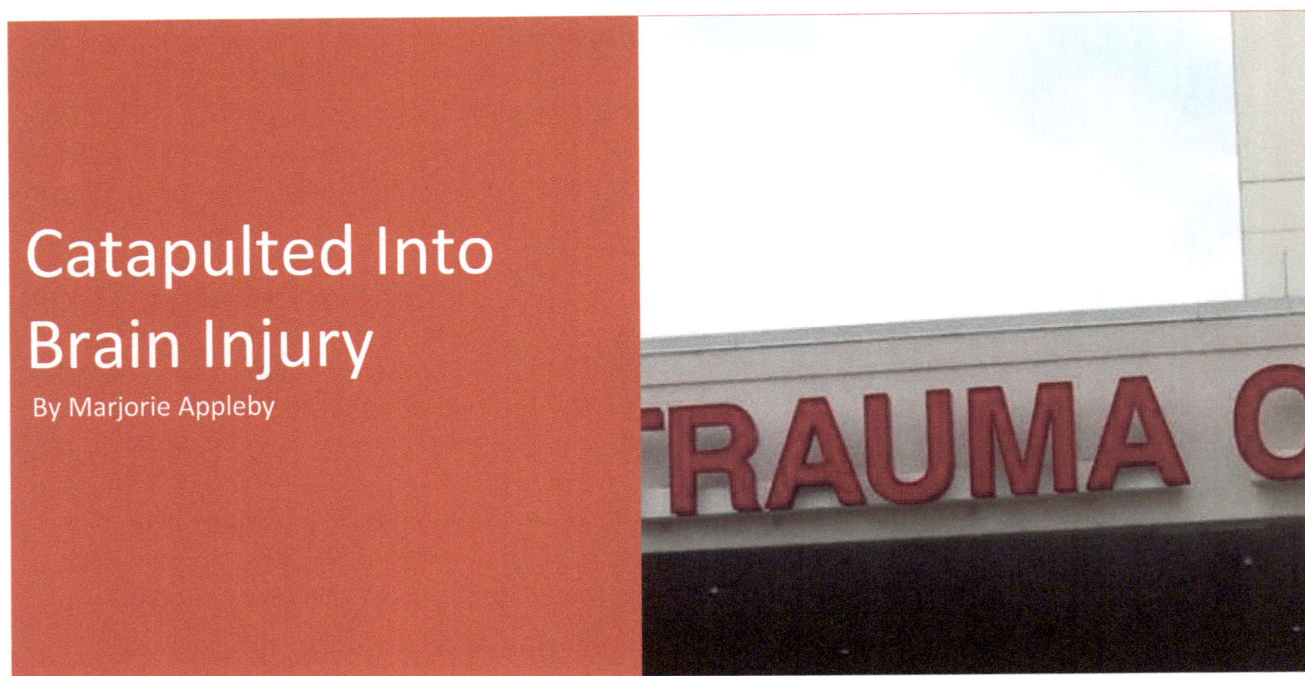

I remember well the event that catapulted our family into the brain injury arena. My son, David, had moved his family to Naples, Florida, a mere twelve days earlier. It was a beautiful Sunday morning when our lives changed in ways we hadn't thought possible. Those who are reading this know exactly what that feels like. We didn't hear the sirens, nor the helicopter that swooped in to take David to the nearest trauma center after he fell out of a vehicle. As the hours passed, we banded together as a family, numb in the realization that the next seventy-two hours would determine whether he would live or die.

Once we knew David was out of immediate danger, the long journey back home began. It was during that time when well-wishing friends and family began to send us information about brain injury, some I put aside to deal with later. Then there were the packages from the Florida Brain and Spinal Cord Injury Program and the Brain Injury Association of Florida, plus the abundance of medical invoices that are part of any medical issue.

> "We didn't hear the sirens, nor the helicopter that swooped in to take David to the nearest trauma center after he fell out of a vehicle."

Since that time, we have struggled with several issues, and as it turns out, we were not alone. We needed something else, besides physical, occupational, and speech therapy. After a full year of helping David to recover from his Traumatic Brain Injury and finding a house to purchase in Naples, a search brought me to a website for survivors and caregivers called Miracles Among Us, Inc. The details are a little fuzzy, but I recall submitting my contact information and waiting to hear from them. Within a week, the founder of Miracles Among Us, Suzan Berg, welcomed us to the community and began to ask questions; how could she help? What could she do to offer us support?

Would we consider driving to Fort Myers, where a Center for Independent Living held a support group meeting? We would meet others who had experienced different types of brain injury.

This started us on our journey of understanding what it was like for David as he has a condition associated with his brain injury called Expressive Aphasia, was in a wheelchair, and often 'zoned out.' We met Jessica that day, a young woman who had experienced a TBI who was open and willing to share what happened to her. I credit Jessica and this group by helping me to understand what was going on within David's mind. This support group has helped to reassure me that there is hope in abundance by enabling me to understand my son in ways he cannot articulate. I am grateful for this opportunity to tell the world of this significant and community-driven organization.

Fast-forward thirteen years, and David is no longer in a wheelchair and strives to achieve at least 10,000 steps using his step-counter. He is by no means the person he once was, but he does participate with our Annual Brain Fair that Miracles Among Us, Inc. organizes during the National Brain Injury month of March. One of our sponsors is the S. Regional Collier County Library, which opens their community room for our free event. All of our Board Members actively seek sponsors and vendors which are healthcare and medical professionals, as well as speakers who bring up-to-date information to share such topics as:

> **"Fast-forward thirteen years, and David is no longer in a wheelchair and strives to achieve at least 10,000 steps using his step-counter."**

- How audio affects the brain
- How to maintain and keep a balanced diet
- Using the correct stimulation
- A myriad of issues specifically for anyone with a brain injury that includes: acquired brain injury, aneurysm, concussion, epilepsy, stroke, and traumatic brain injury

Support groups are formed to allow people to discuss their issues in a safe and friendly, non-judgmental way. Since there was no other support group in the Naples area, Miracles Among Us was incorporated as a 503(c) non-profit organization that conducts a monthly two-hour meeting explicitly designed for survivors and their caregivers of any brain injury.

Our monthly support group also has an appropriate topic to discuss, where the facilitators encourage those who may be reluctant to share. It's a way for them to participate. We often go off-topic, which usually turns out to be a golden nugget. Many will agree that we come away from every meeting with a positive and encouraging feeling. After the meeting, Board Members are often delayed by those who step forward to say our topic was spot-on, and it made a positive impact on their lives. They were glad they made an effort to come.

Most of our members know first-hand that it isn't easy living with a person with brain injury, nor is it effortless to be the survivor. As a group, we strive to cover all aspects of brain injury, including caring for that person. We laugh, we cry, and we sometimes go off-topic. When we begin to doubt ourselves, we tell our members to remember how far they have come from the brink of trauma. We encourage permission to recognize those obstacles that they had to jump over because all of those battles are triumphs.

Anyone who has been through brain injury comes out the other side a changed person, but you should pat yourself on the back. You've come a long, long way, but it was worth it, especially when you share your optimism with others, which in turn gives others hope.

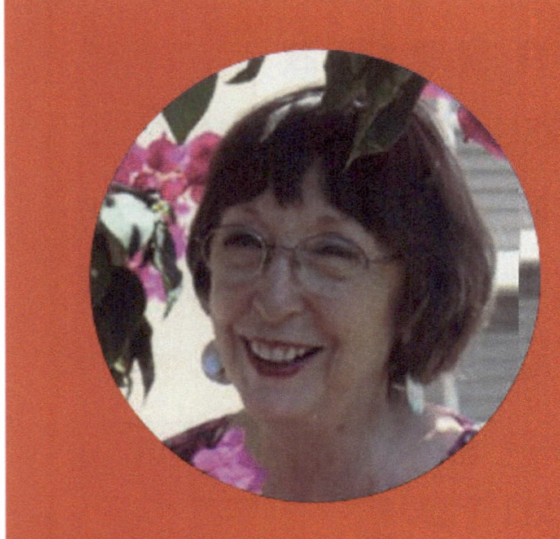

Meet Marjorie Appleby

Marjorie is a National Award-Winning Author with a diversified background that includes Youth Coordinator & Sunday School Teacher, Artist, Author, Certified Landscape Designer, Master Gardener, as well as a 24/7 Caregiver. Her book, RAISING DAVID AGAIN, began as a journal she started the day of her son's accident. As a Brain Injury Advocate, she presents Living With Brain Injury that has been given in Florida and Ohio to caregiver and survivor groups. Marjorie's blog can be found on her website: www.maappleby.com

Living With Hope

By Patrick Brigham

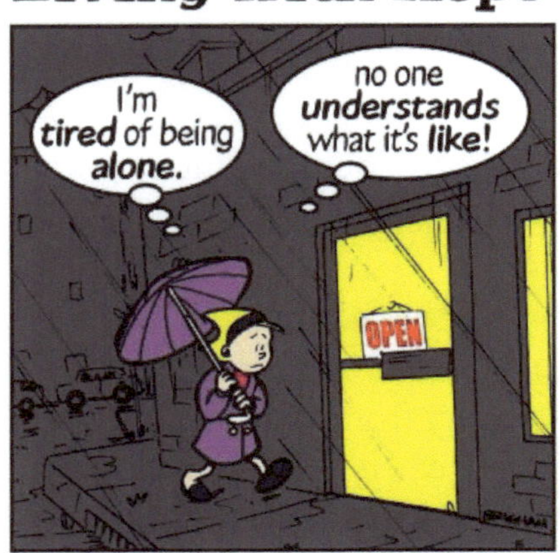

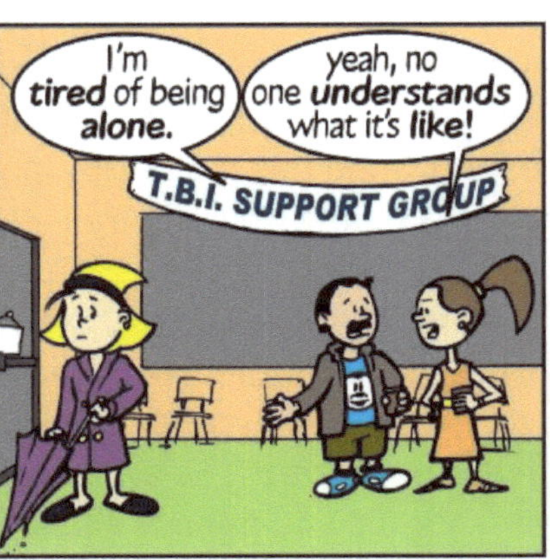

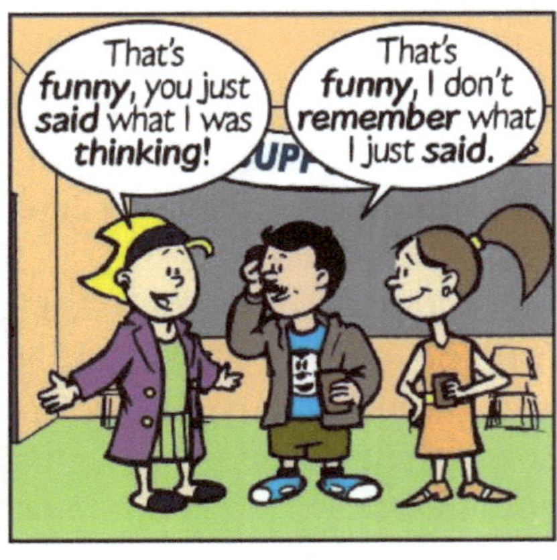

The Blessings of Shared Burdens in Brain Injury

By Nancy Hueber

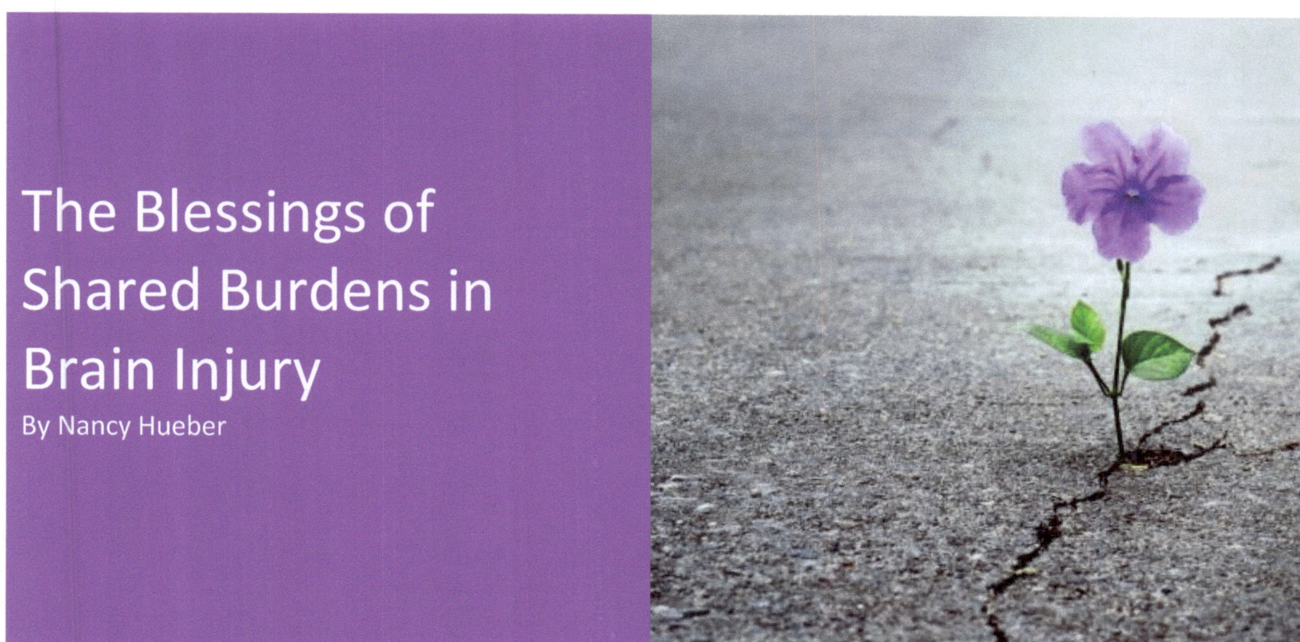

When my husband and I left a Missouri hospital following my brain tumor removal in July of 1996, we had no idea what to expect in the days, weeks and months ahead, let alone years. I could talk and eat, read, hold and play with our three-year-old daughter, and even walk around my block ten days after my craniotomy to remove a near baseball-sized meningioma (non-cancerous) from the middle of my brain. We were relieved for the improvements of no more headaches, dizziness and blurry vision. Heck, we were relieved that I was alive and functioning at all!

The Internet was in its infant stages back in '96, and we bought our first computer the following year in 1997. All that I could find online about my type of brain tumor and possible types of brain injury were medical journal articles with very large words which might as well have said

> "I felt very alone in the company of everyone else who hadn't experienced what I had—a life-changing trauma which had altered me in ways I could never imagine."

"supercalifragilisticexpialidocious" for what I could make out of them. I felt very alone in the company of everyone else who hadn't experienced what I had—a life-changing trauma which had altered me in ways I could never imagine. Where was the help and support I so much needed as everyday life went back to full swing in a world where I felt so much slower?

After the first four years post-brain surgery, I gave birth to our son. As I raised our kids, I noticed more changes in myself which I and my family kept excusing such as memory trouble, bumping into things constantly, having trouble following a recipe or setting out the right number of plates on the table. I had already confronted my left hand difficulties at the piano after thirty-five years of playing and performing, but these everyday issues of injury to my cognitive "executive function" of the brain had not been addressed.

By 2011, I had discovered much more help on the Internet for brain injured people, and I became convinced of the great encouragement which others could find through support groups. I knew that the power of face-to-face support would be extremely powerful in the healing process if I could find a way to connect the dots between others with brain injury in our relatively small Missouri town who were also struggling with their "new normal," a compromised brain affecting them and their families and friends in profound ways.

Could I begin a support group for brain tumor survivors in a town of 25,000? Probably not. Was I brain-injured? Definitely. I decided through much prayer and in discussion with my husband Tom that the more practical route to take in establishing a support group was to make a broader category for all kinds of brain injury survivors and their caregivers.

The first step I took to establish a support group was to go to the local neurologist in our town and ask his office staff if they knew of any support group for their patients. They did not.

Having read books and articles on brain injury over the years, I became more and more certain that a local support group could have a tremendous impact on families who had gone through the brain injury battle or were at the very beginning of the fight to survive all of the unknowns and surprises on their journey. I called Barbara Webster, (whose articles I had read on www.brainline.org) a coordinator of brain injury support groups in Massachusetts, and we talked through how Tom and I could make a brain injury support group happen in our town. Ideas flooded my mind of creating posters to hang across town in physical therapy and medical offices, hospital, drugstores, and even restaurants and schools.

> **"The first step I took to establish a support group was to go to the local neurologist in our town and ask his office staff if they knew of any support group for their patients. They did not."**

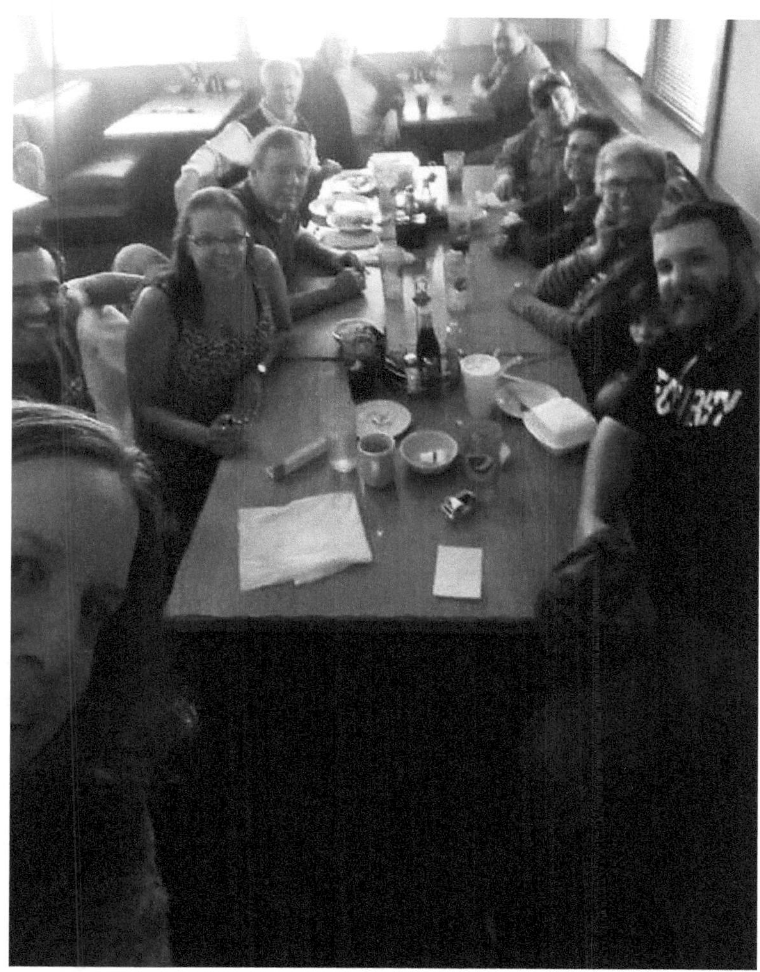

I had met several people and their families who were already facing the struggles of brain injury, so I began to send out invitations with e-mails and phone calls, as well as to establish a meeting place in one of the local churches. And away we went in November of 2012 with monthly (first Monday of the month) meetings filled with tears and laughter, snacks and questions. "What do you do about…" "I'm tired ALL of the time." "ME TOO!" "I like this night light and I have one for each of you to try." "Thanks, Dave!"

We had childcare provided in our first couple of years by a generous hospice volunteer. We mourned over the painful loss of some of our brain cancer survivors who eventually lost their long-fought battles. We rejoiced over the teens who survived horrific car crashes and watched their slow but steady comebacks. We had wonderful dialogues among the caregivers who benefitted from sharing with each other the difficulties of their "new normal," but also heard similar struggles out of other survivors beside their own loved ones.

Sometimes we invited our children to the circle of support to hear from them and vice versa. Our kids became friends who understood their own plights of having a brain-injured parent. We gathered in parks and quiet corners or side rooms of restaurants, enjoyed information-packed presentations by local therapists, doctors or professors, and sometimes the presenters would sit in for our sharing of struggles over the past month. It was important for us to know they were listening to the day-in, day-out issues of brain injury, insurance problems, medication issues, etc. Above all, our local brain injury support group created a space and a "family" to join where we were no longer alone, strange, isolated from the fast-paced world full of bright fluorescent lights (we carried in lamps each month) and quick chatter. We found community, encouragement in identifying so well with each other, learned strategies for daily living from our experiences, talked medicines, doctor recommendations, family dynamics and we made precious friendships.

Eventually, my husband and I had our group become affiliated with the Brain Injury Association of Missouri and shared conference calls with other chapter facilitators. We were supplied posters and other forms of support through the BIA-MO and had visits to our group from the state director. The group very quickly averaged 20-25 attendees monthly and is still going strong seven years later! We moved in 2016 out-of-state, but by then, the BIA-MO chapter in our town had become a nurturing and welcoming place of support. New leaders from the group stepped up to the plate and provided the necessary communications and direction which that group will always need, in addition to their understanding and love.

Although I received and still enjoy giving and receiving support online, I know that my husband and I would both say that the physical presence of a local support group provides incredible face-to-face support; it may lead to lifelong friendships and activities together (yes, we even tried bowling) and to have the opportunity to build one another up in a compassionate and brave way after brain injury!

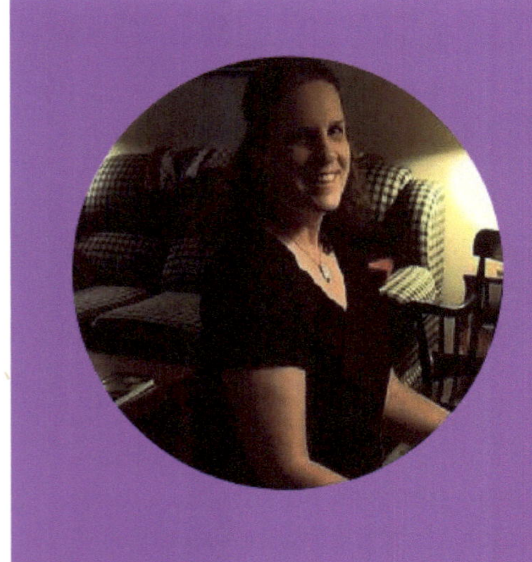

Meet Nancy Hueber

Nancy Hueber, a professional pianist, wife, mother, and frequent visitor to her couch and bed, survived a near baseball-sized brain tumor (meningioma) in the middle of her brain, and its removal by craniotomy six days later. In 2012, Nancy and her husband Tom established a brain injury support group in their town in northeast Missouri, now affiliated with the Brain Injury Association of Missouri. Their monthly meetings are attended by both brain injury survivors and their caregivers, with injuries received from brain tumors, strokes, aneurysms, accidents and/or concussions.

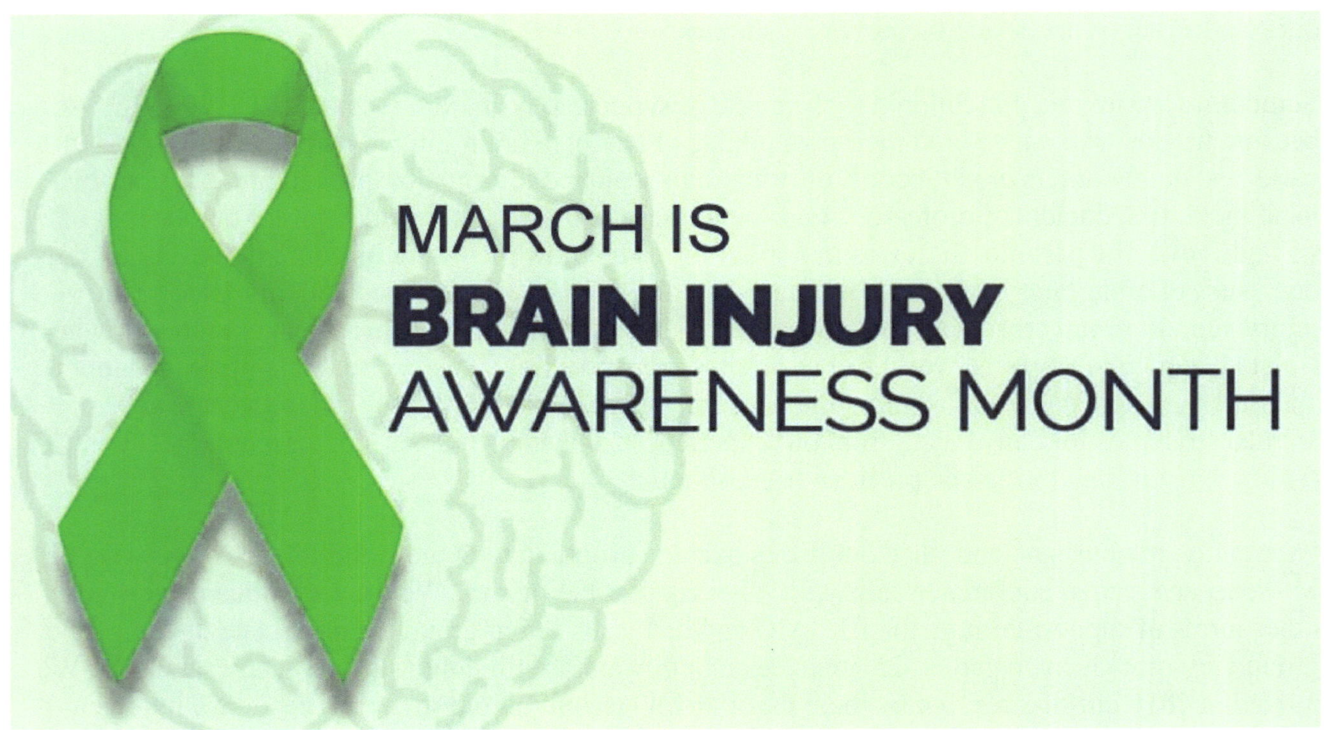

Shelter From The Storm

By Ric Johnson

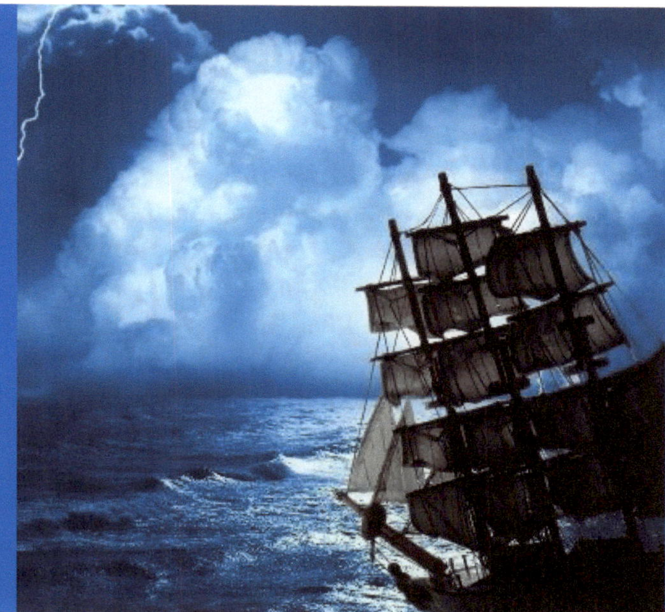

I became a brain injury survivor in October 2003 after I fell from a ladder and hit my head on a concrete slab on my driveway. U then spent my first month in a medically induced coma after a craniology surgery. My second and third months were spent in two different hospitals for cognitive and speech therapy. In January 2004, I was released from the hospital and sent home, but continued with speech and occupational therapy as an out-patient in a local rehabilitation center. After nine months, I graduated from my therapy sessions and was told that the rehab center had a support group that I should attend.

All I could think about was, "What? A support group? I don't need a 12 Step program. I'm fully aware of my injury and accept my difficulties. In July 2011, I was at the rehab center for a different event and read a poster about their brain injury support group. For some reason, that really clicked and seemed to be important. I checked my calendar, and my night was free on their next meeting. As that date came closer, I kept thinking that attending was more than important. Walking into that meeting was daunting. All I could think about was, "what would they ask me to do?" "Would I need to prove that I'm a TBI survivor?" "Would there be dues to pay?" "I'm alone, my wife can't come, what the heck am I'm doing?" Even so, I walked in, and have never regretted it.

> "As the meeting started, I was told there is a rule when a "new" person attends a meeting, that other members would introduce themselves and gave a short story concerning their injury first."

The facilitator saw me, dropped her conversation with another person, walked up, introduced herself and welcomed me. I looked around, didn't see a person I knew, and was trying to figure out where to sit when another member of the group said, "this chair is open," and she held out her hand as a friend.

As the meeting started, I was told there is a rule when a "new" person attends a meeting, that other members would introduce themselves and give a short story concerning their injury. I was also told I didn't need to say a thing unless I wanted too when they were done.

The first thought that came to my head as they were talking was, holy cow I am not alone. I heard them talk about the same problems I had or still have, the same techniques that did or did not help my recovery, and the same daily problems or gains. When it was my time, I did talk. My name, my injury, my fears, my PTSD, my why, why, why. As I talked, I saw many smiles, a lot of nods, and a lot of yep, yep and yep. I had never met a survivor before, but during that meeting I understood that even though my injury maybe different from other survivors, I am one of many. I was so impressed I was sorry when we closed up. A month later, I was there again. Then the month after that. In fact, I haven't missed a meeting for eight years unless I'm out of town.

A support group allows survivors and family members to meet face-to-face with others in the same position they find themselves in. A support group meeting is not a private therapy session. The goal is to share strategies, techniques and tips to help everyone navigating into a world the survivor did not expect to live in or plan for.

As we become aware of our injury, we hear something called the New Normal. In the local support group I attend, we call it the Current Normal. We also say that recovery never stops, as long as we do not stop. Of course, we cannot undo our injury, but we can try to make sure that we do not have another brain injury by following those tips or strategies shared by other survivors.

Is a face-to-face support group meeting better than an on-line forum or Facebook page? In my opinion, yes. Since every person is different, so are brain injuries. Each grieving process is different. Each recovery process is different. Each person's ability to sit in a room with unfamiliar people, with different noises or lighting, with different emotions, with different expectations differs. Each meeting is a give and take process. We can give new survivors, and their families, an insight that took us years to understand all the wins we won against our daily battles.

At meetings we hear phrases like, "How long does it take for my short-term memory to get better?," "How long does to take for my friends to understand me?" or "Why doesn't my doctor believe me?" There are no easy answers for those questions, but we can help people understand that the key to getting more good days then bad days is all

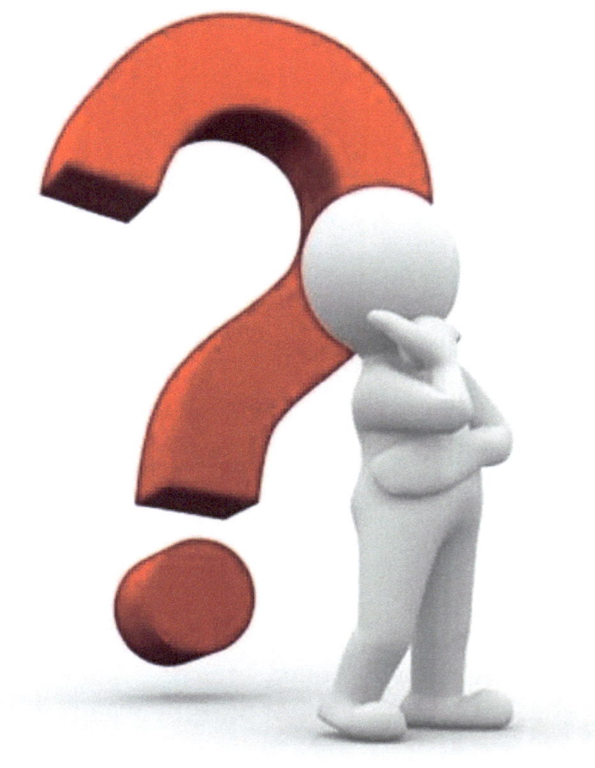

about perception. When members tell us they did something that surprised them, we give them a shout of congratulations.

It's not unusual for some members to arrive and almost never say a thing, but they are there to listen. They know that what happens, or said, in a meeting stays in the meeting. They know that nobody judges anyone. Sometimes the meetings will have a guest speaker, maybe a music or art therapist, an author, but most often a topic that gets people thinking out-of-the box and they ask for that topic to be on the next month's agenda.

Today I am the facilitator for the support group I first went to eight years ago. I didn't boss my way into removing the facilitator before me, she moved away and asked me and another person to take her place. I could not be more pleased. Helping others and having others help me, will make sure my recovery will never be done/finished/completed. If you know there is a support group near you, but never attended, give it a chance. You will not be sorry.

To paraphrase a poet, support groups are created to give survivors "shelter from the storm."

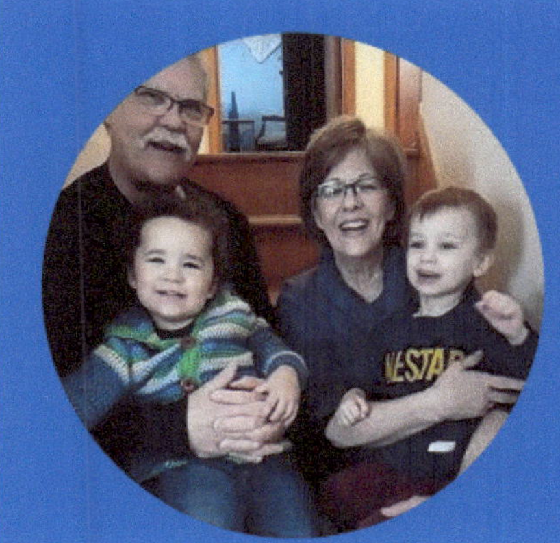

Meet Ric Johnson

Ric Johnson is a husband, father, and grandfather. A survivor from a traumatic brain injury of 15+ years. Ric is also a member of the Speaker Bureau for the Minnesota Brain Injury Alliance, and facilitator for The Courage Kenny Brain Injury Support Group.

Brain Injury
Affects the Entire Family.

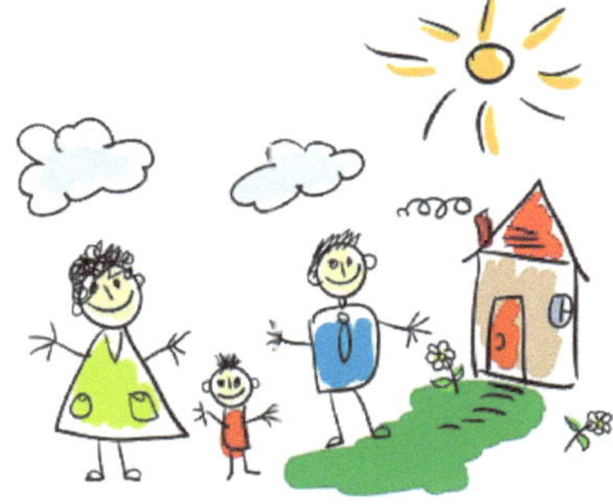

Good Grief

By Debra Gorman

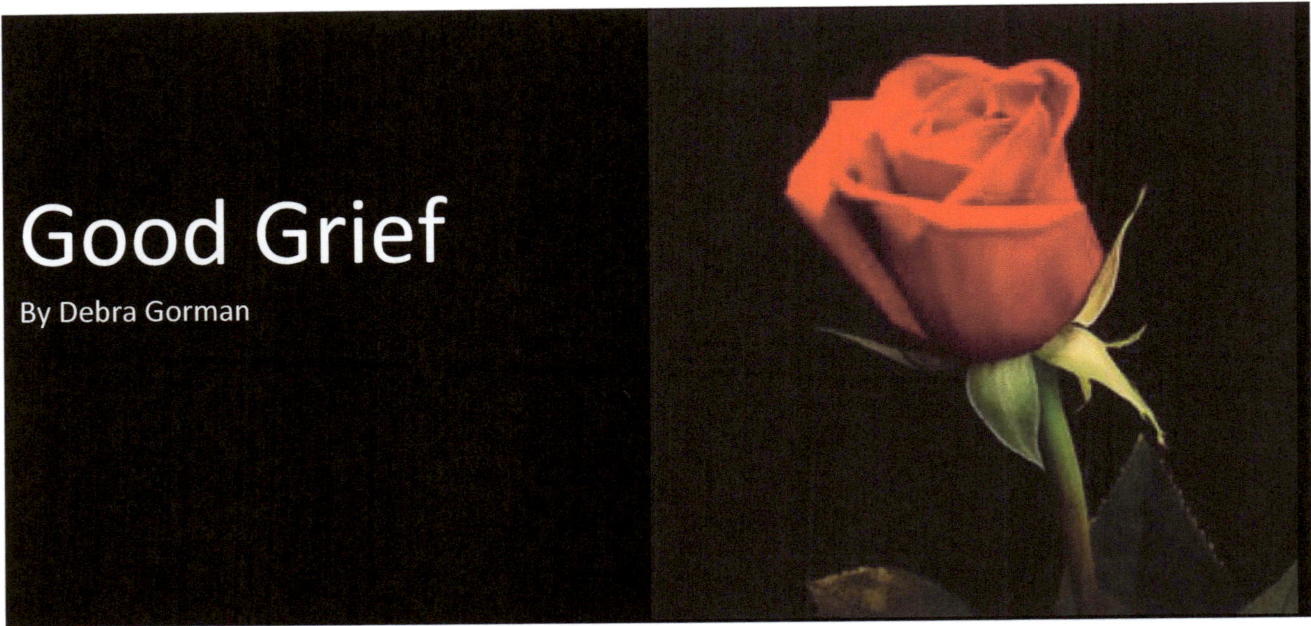

I started looking for a grief support group when it became clear that I would not fully recover from my brain hemorrhage. My new self was so burdensome, so uncomfortable. I dreamed of having a ten minute reprieve, just ten minutes to feel like I used to feel, to be how I used to be. It was so much work being me now. I missed my former self terribly. To be honest, I was a little ashamed of the new me. I didn't like standing out in a negative way, of being "different." In the past I had always made sure my appearance was good, even if life was falling apart around me. Now, balance and walking was difficult and awkward. I suffered unusual fatigue.

> "Whether your experience is loss of health, loss of a job, a divorce, death, you name it. The grieving process is basically the same. Loss is loss. Grief is grief."

My hormones, which are regulated in the brain, stopped working and I put on a lot of weight. I felt unattractive and feared loved ones would stop loving me. I struggled mightily for improvement. It was eight years ago when my brain spontaneously bled, and frankly, I haven't advanced very much since that time. I'm simply learning to adapt. I have sporadically searched for a group to support loss for nearly eight years.

The groups I found were for people who had experienced the death of someone close. Well, who is closer to you than you? The groups I found were not for someone like me, although I have experienced tremendous losses in my life, starting in childhood. Whether your experience is loss of health, loss of a job, a divorce, death, you name it, the grieving process is basically the same. Loss is loss. Grief is grief.

I have found that well-meaning people can say very hurtful things. For example, "I thought you'd be over it by now." "There must be a reason." "It could have been worse." Although those statements may contain an element of truth, they are totally unhelpful. What I needed was to express my sorrow and be heard, without judgement. I started reading about grief and studying it. I found comfort and validation. A book written by Doug Manning, an expert in grief counseling, wrote about grief: "The path is not smooth or even well marked." In my mind I drifted back in time. I used to do a lot of hiking and backpacking on the Fingerlakes Trail in upstate New York where I lived. The trail is marked by painted white brushstrokes on the trunks of trees, or white plastic rectangles of about equal size nailed to trees. Some trails were well marked with abundant blazes to show the way. Other sections of the same trail had few signs, making it difficult to stay on the correct path. To make matters worse, there were plenty of times when I had my head down, taking care not to stumble, or I was lost in thought, only to look up and discover that I was truly lost.

I learned that one does not rise through grief in a steady upward fashion. It has been described as waves that keep coming and they wash over you. Occasionally, at unexpected, inconvenient times they will rush at you and knock you down. Also, grief will find expression in one way or another. In order to access healthy grieving, it may help to schedule time for reflection and tears. You may want the experience to be private, but it can also be beneficial to have a trusted person with you, someone who knows the ground rules: don't try to fix it. There may be tears and "why" questions, and that is okay.

I have learned that grief never completely resolves. If you had a child who died, would you ever stop missing that child? At best, I think you learn to live with grief, to adapt to it, to make room for it in your life. Grief changes you forever, and since we can't change the event that caused the grief, we can find purpose in it. We can be the person who comes alongside someone else. We can listen without judgement or trying to repair the person.

I'm thinking grief is like hiking an unfamiliar, difficult trail with plenty of switchbacks and elevation changes. You may have a guide, someone who knows the path and can lead the way, or you may bushwhack your way through the density, with little more than a compass in your toolkit. Eventually, you can arrive at the same place, but no one else can do the work. You must shoulder your pack and push ahead, no matter how much your body and your heart aches. Usually, at some unknowable point in time, you will come out on the other side.

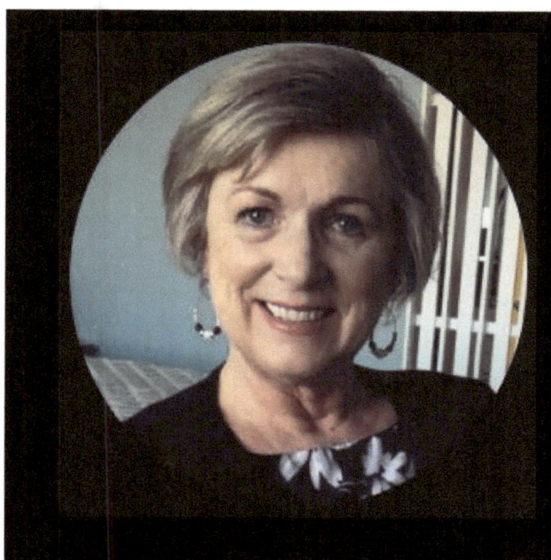

Meet Debra Gorman

Debra Gorman was fifty-six years old in 2011 when she experienced a cavernous angioma on her brain stem, causing her brain to bleed. Four months later she sustained a subdural hematoma. She later learned that she also had suffered a stroke during one of those events. She had been married only six years to her beloved. Debra considers what she has priceless: the love and support of her husband, children and friends. For many years she has written for her blog, entitled Graceful Journey. debralynn48.wordpress.com

News & Views

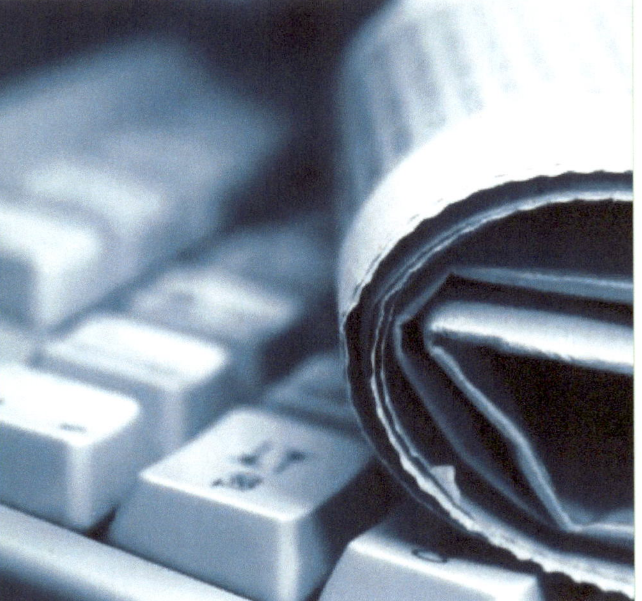

News & Views

By David & Sarah Grant

The past few weeks have been filled with uncertainty and concern for all of us. We've been notified of several annual Brain Injury Conferences have been cancelled due to the recent coronavirus outbreak. Conferences help so many within the brain injury community and offer the ability for many of us to come together as a true community in a face-to-face environment. Over the last ten years, some of our fondest memories have come from brain injury conferences.

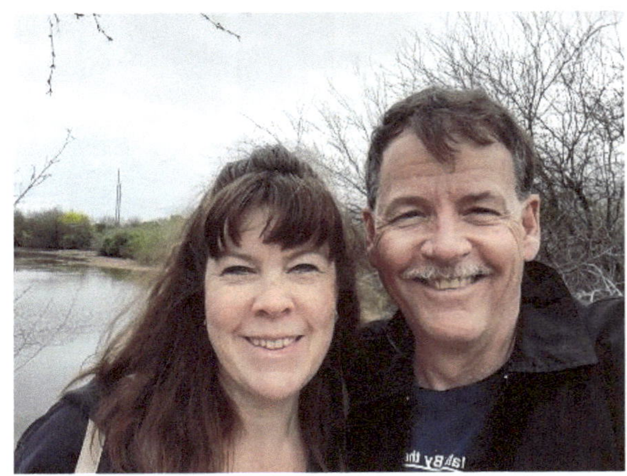

But these days, our common welfare comes first. Being mindful of health is not just something important to us within the brain injury family, it is a common denominator for all humanity.

It's a reasonable bet that the uncertainly will continue for a while. As social gatherings are already being scaled back, brain injury support groups are already being affected. We encourage you to use this time as a unique opportunity to serve others. A phone call to a survivor or family member, just letting them know that they are in your thoughts, can do wonders to help ease anxiety. An email or text only takes a minute or two and can change the course of someone's day.

With as much conflicting information as there is right now, we are sticking to basics – frequent hand-washing, social distancing, and simply using good common sense. When brain injury became part of our lives, we learned that together we can walk through just about anything. This will be no different.

Peace,

~ David & Sarah